The Rise of Autism

This innovative book addresses the question of why increasing numbers of people are being diagnosed with autism since the 1990s. Providing an engaging account of competing and widely debated explanations, it investigates how these have led to differing interpretations of the same data. Crucially, the author argues that the increased use of autism diagnosis is due to medicalisation across the life course, whilst holding open the possibility that the rise may also be partly accounted for by modern-day environmental exposures, again, across the life course.

A further focus of the book is *not* on whether autism itself is valid as a diagnostic category, but whether and how it is useful as a diagnostic category, and how the utility of the diagnosis has contributed to the rise. This serves to move beyond the question of whether diagnoses are 'real' or social constructions, and instead asks: who do diagnoses serve to benefit, and at what cost do they come?

The book will appeal to clinicians and health professionals, as well as medical researchers, who are interested in a review of the data which demonstrates the rising use of autism as a diagnosis, and an analysis of the reasons why this has occurred. Providing theory through which to interpret the expanding application of the diagnosis and the broadening of autism as a concept, it will also be of interest to scholars and students of sociology, philosophy, psychiatry, psychology, social work, disability studies and childhood studies.

Ginny Russell is Senior Lecturer at the University of Exeter, in the UK. She co-leads the Health and Illness theme at Egenis (the Centre for the Study of Life Sciences) in the College of Social Science and International Studies, as well as co-leading the Epidemiology and Qualitative Research stream of ChYMe (the Children and Young People's Mental Health collaboration) based at the College of Medicine and Health.

Routledge Studies in the Sociology of Health and Illness

For more information about this series, please visit: www.routledge.com/
Routledge-Studies-in-the-Sociology-of-Health-and-Illness/book-series/RSSHI

The Rise of Autism

Risk and Resistance in the
Age of Diagnosis

Ginny Russell

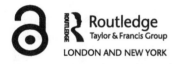

Routledge
Taylor & Francis Group

LONDON AND NEW YORK

First published 2021
by Routledge
2 Park Square, Milton Park, Abingdon, Oxon OX14 4RN

and by Routledge
605 Third Avenue, New York, NY 10158

Routledge is an imprint of the Taylor & Francis Group, an informa business

Cover art work by J.A. Tan. Find more of J.A. Tan's work at the-art-of-autism.com,
and artofjatan.com

Trademark notice: Product or corporate names may be trademarks or registered trademarks,
and are used only for identification and explanation without intent to infringe.

British Library Cataloguing-in-Publication Data
A catalogue record for this book is available from the British Library

Library of Congress Cataloging-in-Publication Data
Names: Russell, Ginny, 1965– author.
Title: The rise of autism: risk and resistance in the age of diagnosis / Ginny Russell.
Description: Milton Park, Abingdon, Oxon; New York, NY: Routledge, 2021. |
Series: Routledge studies in the sociology of health and illness |
Includes bibliographical references and index.
Identifiers: LCCN 2020039810 (print) | LCCN 2020039811 (ebook) |
ISBN 9780367250812 (hardback) | ISBN 9780429285912 (ebook)
Subjects: LCSH: Autism. | Autism–Diagnosis. | Autism–Environmental aspects.
Classification: LCC RC553.A88 R87 2021 (print) |
LCC RC553.A88 (ebook) | DDC 616.85/882–dc23
LC record available at https://lccn.loc.gov/2020039810
LC ebook record available at https://lccn.loc.gov/2020039811

ISBN: 978-0-367-25081-2 (hbk)
ISBN: 978-0-367-69546-0 (pbk)
ISBN: 978-0-429-28591-2 (ebk)

Typeset in Galliard
by Newgen Publishing UK

For Susan Kelly

Contents

Illustrations

Figures

Tables

Acknowledgements

This work was generously funded by the Wellcome Trust as part of an Investigator Award, *Exploring Diagnosis*, grant number 108676/Z/15/Z SfZ. I would like to thank the Ex Dx team, my collaborators on all the studies and the PhD students from whom I have learnt so much: Abby Russell, Selina Nath, Jennie Hayes, Tom Lister, Victoria Wren, Elena Sharratt and Rhianna White, as well as people who were kind enough to read draft chapters: Annemarie Jutel, Stuart Logan, Mike Michael, Peter Carpenter, Christine Hauskeller, Ilina Singh, Delphine Jacobs, Su Lovell, Virginia Bovell, Katherine Runswick-Cole, Adam Feinstein and Steven Kapp. Thanks also to JA Tan for the cover art, Ann Grand for edits and James Vine for designing the fabulous graphics.

Introduction

Autism is being diagnosed more often in both children and adults. The big question is *why?*

This book aims to answer that question by offering an account of the modern-day (post-1990) rise in the use of autism as a diagnosis. My research in this topic comes from my work as an epidemiologist and social scientist with a strong interest in the activist counter-narrative of neurodiversity.[1] My view is partial and situated;[2] my knowledge spans both the above disciplines but does neither of them justice. Therefore, I have chosen to address this question with a focus on what I do know about: my research, which has led me to reflect on how the work was carried out, who shaped it and why. The book focuses on my research in the last ten years, much of which has been carried out in collaboration with various colleagues and students; some of the empirical work reported here is new and some comes from published studies.

The post-1990 period has been a time of change and, in high-income countries, roughly equates to the period sociologists refer to as late modernity;[3] a time in which identity politics and self-definition have intensified. This has in turn shaped medicine, particularly in the field of autism research. I hope this book will reflect this and be read not only by academics and clinicians but also by people with autism/autistic people (I will be using these two terms interchangeably[i]) as well as people in autism-related jobs, educators, health professionals, students and parents of people with autism.

The rise in autism diagnoses since the 1990s is a phenomenon of high-income countries, particularly those in North America and Europe. We have no reliable data to identify trends in autism diagnosis for lower- and middle-income countries. According to our cross-sectional review of published papers in autism research in 2016,[4] we found (but had no space to report) that 85% of autism research took place in North America and Europe, and 45% of European research happened in the UK (Figure I.1). Very little research (<1%) originated from

---

i The terms are used interchangeably in this book, as 'person with autism' is used in psychiatric epidemiological literature, whereas 'autistic' is preferred by activists in the autism community. Chapter 4 gives an account of this position.

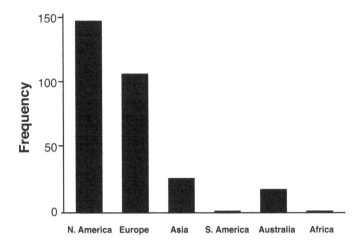

Figure I.1 Distribution of autism studies by continent from cross-sectional review. Includes all autism research studies published in top four autism-specific journals in 2016.

either Africa or South America. There is just not enough data from lower-income countries to analyse time trends.

In addition, many low- and middle-income countries, including much of Asia and most of Africa, still consider autism to be a condition that was almost always associated with an intellectual disability. In the UK and USA, autism is increasingly being diagnosed in children with above-average intelligence (Chapter 3 covers the implications of this). The trend of autism diagnosis in various low- and middle-income countries may be very different to that in Europe and North America.

Why is autism on the rise?

The trend of increasing diagnosis of autism since 1990 is established in Chapter 1, with data from many settings. The reasons for the upsurge in diagnosis are hotly debated. Some researchers attribute the rise solely to *artefactual*, not actual, increases and others suspect the rise is both artefactual and *real*; in other words there are more children with autistic-type behaviours around today than there were in 1990.

The *artefactual* account of the increased use of autism diagnosis is partly due to the medicalisation of behaviour at the milder end of the spectrum to bring it under the banner of 'diagnosable autism': changes in methods of identification, diagnostic substitution, increased awareness, shifts in understanding, together resulting in the broadening use of the label. All these things have prompted increased diagnosis, as many excellent historical and sociological texts have shown.[5-9] This book concentrates on another mechanism, the increased diagnosis and recording of autism in new cohorts of people, babies, infants, children, adults, even dead people: divided by stages across the life course.

Many parents, activists, clinicians and researchers believe that there is a *real* rise in autism, as our study, reported in Chapter 7, attests. By 'real' I mean that a larger percentage of the population has severe autistic symptoms[ii] than in previous generations. In Part II, I'll hold open, and attempt to consider some of the evidence for, the possibility that the rise may be fuelled or partly accounted for by modern social trends, changes in medical practices or environmental exposures. In this account, there is an increased risk of autism because some novel environmental, medical (for example, a new drug used in pregnancy) or social trigger (such as older parenthood) disturbs neurodevelopment. Risk factors such as these might also be associated with more cases of a range of neurodevelopmental problems, leading to outcomes such as intellectual disability, attention deficit hyperactivity disorder (ADHD), language delay or disrupted neurodevelopment across the board, so a broad view is adopted.

The general consensus in mainstream autism science, among epidemiologists and most autism researchers, is that the rise in the use of a diagnosis of autism diagnosis is artefactual.[10] In Chapters 2–6, I will describe how autism diagnosis (or pre-diagnosis) has been extended to types of people it was almost never applied to before 1990. The rise itself has contributed to increased awareness – a form of looping:[11] the rise prompts more awareness which in turn fuels the rise. Such looping effects are brilliantly described in Ethan Watters's book *Crazy Like Us*.[12] He demonstrates how Western psychiatric categories, such as anorexia, depression and post-traumatic stress disorder, have been relentlessly publicised in Asia, leading to huge apparent jumps in prevalence in Asian countries. Also, services directed at autism and the availability of diagnostic assessment bolster the rates of diagnosis. I will give examples of some other forms of looping effects, as well as discussing pertinent modern narratives in autism research that have effectively fuelled autism's rise.

The debate over how to account for the rise – whether it is entirely artefactual, or whether it is both artefactual *and* real – is a touchstone of this book, seeking to move beyond the somewhat tired question of whether diagnoses are 'true' neurodevelopmental differences or social constructions (they are both) to ask, in conclusion, who benefits from autism diagnoses? And at what cost? Is autism *useful* as a diagnostic category and if so, for whom, when and under what circumstances?

As a diagnosis, autism has many functions: for clinicians, to organise treatment, services and predict outcomes; for insurance companies, to process payments; for researchers, as a way to organise the field; for activists, as a banner to rally beneath; for lawyers, as a way to decide who is responsible for their actions.[13] But it is also crucial for parents or for autistic adults, in terms of gaining access to services, rewriting biography and providing an explanatory frame, giving meaning.

---

ii Symptoms is a word that is also contested in relation to autism but is used in psychiatric epidemiological literature; it is objectionable to wave 2 thinkers because it positions autism as akin to disease.

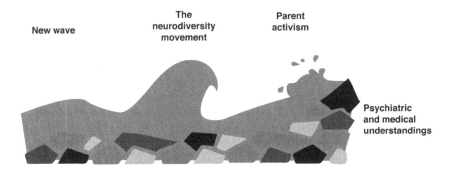

Figure I.2 Waves of autism activism.

More sinister is the benefit for Autism Inc., the chain of professionalisation and commercialisation that runs in parallel with the rising use of diagnosis.

Tribes

Autism has inspired a huge amount of 'tribal' community, political and social activism over many decades,[14] as described in Steve Silberman's book *Neurotribes*. Three 'tribal' viewpoints of autism can be broadly and briefly characterised[15–17] as occurring in waves (Figure I.2), each in reaction against and resistance to the previous conceptualisation. Diagnosis positions autism as a disorder but how people regard diagnosis reflects the waves of autism research and activism. The bedrock of medical and psychiatric understanding slowly erodes as the waves lift and lash against it and in turn, the shape of the bedrock alters the waves.

The understanding of clinical, epidemiological and biomedical scientists in the autism research community was originally that autism was triggered by cold parenting and should be diagnosed using the expertise of psychiatry. Today, scientists believe that autism is a neurodevelopmental disorder that encompasses a spectrum of differences and should be diagnosed using the shared expertise of psychiatry, clinical psychology or paediatrics. The first wave of resistance, breaking against the dominance of psychiatry in opposition to parent blame, largely prompted by parent activists, was that parents are the real experts. This wave of autism activism developed into one that sees autism as a biochemical neurological condition that clinicians should diagnose, and treat (and cure if possible). This 'pro-cure' wave peaked in the early 2000s. The 'tribe' are mostly parents of severely affected children and speak passionately of the importance of efforts to develop biomedical treatment for a highly impairing and distressing condition that they see as akin to a disease[18] and certainly as a disorder. First-wave thinkers put forward the notion of an autism 'epidemic'[19] whose origin, as argued by fundamentalists in the tribe, was not only biological but environmental, the consequence of new exposures.

Autistic activism emerged in resistance to the risk discourse of the first wave, which painted autism as a threat to be feared and as a tragedy. This wave of thinking is ascendant, and it encompasses a broadly anti-cure stance, led by autistic activists and allies. This wave argued for autism as an identity, an integral and important difference that, although challenging and impairing, should not be cured and regarded not as a tragedy but as a disability. Accommodations to support autistic people to live well should be provided. There are children and adults with real neurodevelopmental differences, sometimes profound differences that cause distressing impairments. But distress is also caused by discrimination which, combined with a lack of adjustment by other members of society, denies them full participation in the world. This wave paved the way for the emergence of the neurodiversity movement and self-identification as autistic. A part of our group's work has been to bring together autistic adults influential in the movement; the authors of a collection put out by Steven Kapp in 2020[1] which, together with Tom Lister's PhD research on self-identification and diagnosis,[20] revealed many engaged adults who firmly consider autism as identity rather than disorder, promoting diagnosis but in a less pathologising frame.

In this context, it is clear why the idea of the real increase, an environmental risk factor that precipitates autism or has a role in increase of autism or autism traits, is understandably problematic for some neurodiversity theorists. The environmental trigger theories of diet, heavy metals and pollution drove the hardcore faction in the first wave, who seemed, to autistic self-advocates, to be intent on eliminating people like them. According to Kapp, himself an autistic activist, arguments against environmental toxins as a risk factor for autism help to 'direct parents away from cottage industries based on rejected and unproven theories that offer dangerous "treatments" like heavy metal-injecting chelation therapy, chemical castration (Lupron therapy) bleach enemas and vaccine avoidance (amid other expensive or at least ill-conceived "interventions")'.[1] Many in the neurodiversity wave reject causal models that implicate environmental exposures not only because they are sceptical of the evidence but also because arguments for rights hinge on neurological differences (meaning neurological structural differences with a genetic origin) that are present from, or even before, birth. One can make an argument for rights based on differences acquired via exposure (wheelchair users need and deserve ramps in the present, regardless of whether they were fully mobile at some point in their lives) but nevertheless, many advocates reject the idea that autism is a result of an injury.

In different ways, the actions of both the neurodiversity advocates and the pro-cure tribe seem to adopt, shore up and dismantle a more medicalised model.[21] Each wave has spawned its own competing language and associated narratives. I hope to draw attention to the use of language in medical and resistance discourse and its influence in constraining the possibilities for thought and action, even though at times I will be using the aforementioned language myself, adopting the conventions of some source texts. The over-arching point is that each 'tribe' has a distinct standpoint on how autism is conceptualised and advocates for autistic people in particular ways. The result is an epistemic battleground, in which each faction claims authority over knowledge of autism. Each wave of thinking has swelled in resistance to what went before, growing through people who care, yet feel silenced and marginalised. Perhaps a new wave is even now brewing.

In high-income countries, the post-1990, late-modern period is associated with a rise in self-characterisation,[3] as opposed to the earlier, traditional modern, period when ordered systems prevailed and people were told what they were. Perhaps this explains the misunderstandings over the third-wave autism-as-an-identity and the traditional view of autism-as-disorder. Proponents of the neurodiversity movement, especially autistic activists, have reclaimed autism for their own since 1990 but autism-as-disorder is still traditionally operationalised by psychiatrists, clinicians and researchers.[22] All parties have epistemic authority but know things in different ways. The tribe of those considered expert has grown to include parents, autistic adults and many types of professionals, all of whom contribute their own ways of defining autism. The result is to multiply the ways in which autism is understood and recognised.

The bio-politics of autism illustrate how the same data can be interpreted in very different ways by different groups to advance their agendas. The politics of autism *are* bio-politics, not in a Foucauldian sense, but because different groups (hybrids of clinicians, self-advocates, parents and researchers) have mobilised around the diagnostic category. They influence how information is disseminated, by whom and why. The 'tribal' stories mesh, or sometimes contrast, with the consensus and narratives of science. A multi-level view of autism, together with a personal reflection that underscores my point, will be found in the conclusion. This will help to answer the guiding question: *why is autism on the rise?*

What is autism?

I was once lucky enough to attend a lecture given by the legendary Sir Michael Rutter, often called the father of modern child psychiatry. A member of the audience asked him, 'what is ADHD?'

This was the wrong question, he replied. ADHD is a diagnostic category like any other; a way of putting a boundary round a collection of signs and symptoms (its 'symptoms' being mostly behaviours). ADHD, he explained, is a useful psychiatric construction but it does not exist separately from the definition that we give it. It does not carve nature at the joints but is a pragmatic response, designed to help children with distressing difficulties. Its boundaries are in a state of slow flux, as our understanding of the behavioural traits that comprise the condition evolve in step with research, expertise and society's demands. This was a striking statement from a leading autism researcher.

Like ADHD, autism can be thought of as a multi-dimensional collection of psychological traits that interact with each other and the environment; traits that may alter with development. These traits are identified from behaviours that recur in multiple settings and at multiple times. They are bound together not only for medical diagnostic reasons but also for historical, pragmatic and political reasons. Figure I.3 is a schematic illustration of how biology underpins

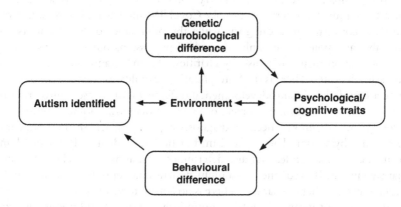

Figure I.3 A model of identification in the clinic.

autism but interacts with social and environmental factors at every level and how in clinical practice autism is identified by pervasive behaviours rather than biological tests. In common with all diseases and disorders, autism is *both* a real neurodevelopmental difference *and* socially framed.

The social construction of autism's boundaries, *vis-à-vis* its neurological actuality, can be illustrated using Covid-19. Like autism, Covid-19, as a disease entity, can be considered an object around which a boundary is placed (although it is unclear whether this qualifies it as a 'boundary object', as described by Leigh Star[23]). In the UK, a person's primary cause of death is categorised by the Office for National Statistics (ONS). The ONS attributes deaths to a discrete cause, usually a disease, such as cancer, dementia or cardiovascular/heart disease. Or Covid-19. The record therefore reports a decision about what that one person died from. Covid-19, or any other disease, is a distinct cause which, from the ONS statisticians' point of view, must be distinguished so that statistical analyses can be carried out. The reality, in many cases, is that a Covid-19 infection affects functioning across multiple biological systems, especially the respiratory system, leaving a person susceptible to underlying health issues. It is plausible some deaths resulted from a tipping over due to unrecognised infection by Covid-19, even if the person were asymptomatic and the infection therefore unidentified; the infection may have undermined the person's defences against their pre-existing conditions, which predisposed their exacerbation. Inversely, underlying conditions may make a person more vulnerable to Covid-19. Elderly people with pre-existing health conditions are the most at risk from Covid-19 infection: pre-existing frailty means vulnerability. People's biological and psychological resilience may also be undermined by the response to Covid-19: the lockdown, social isolation, lack of access to services, and so on. Distinguishing one 'cause' of death is a pragmatic construction, whereas the interaction of biological and social systems being tipped over by infection is closer to reality.

I think autism may be a 'boundary' object, in that there is a reality of neurodevelopmental difference. But like Covid-19, and like most diseases, a continuum is converted to a category, while the boundaries of 'what counts' are permeable and policed, certainly by medical professions but increasingly, since the mobilisation of parents, also by charities, autism organisations and autistic adult self-advocates. There is the 'interpretative flexibility' of a boundary object.[24] There are underlying neurodevelopmental differences, of course, but there is no 'real' or 'not real' autism, no correct or incorrect diagnosis, no misdiagnosis, no under- or over-diagnosis, because diagnosis depends on where the boundaries are set, and by whom. There is autism, but how it is identified, described and classified is a human endeavour and determines what autism looks like. Autism is what we say it is. If we define it as a multi-dimensional set of behavioural traits at a certain severity, that is what it is. There is no autism to be discovered 'out there'. But that does not mean it is not an enormously important and useful construct that describes, and helps meet, impairing and challenging difficulties.

In his response to the question about ADHD, Rutter acknowledged that the group of people who are diagnosed with a condition might change as a slightly different (or expanded) collection of symptoms is identified. When does a collection of symptoms become a diagnosis? Robert Aronowitz[25] draws an analogy with the question of *when does a dialect become a language?* His answer is the well-known quip that a language is a dialect *with an army.* There are many discourses about the signifiers of autism and varying theories of the underlying biological, psychological and social mechanisms that lead to its development. Providing a comprehensive definition of autism is problematic. Autism inevitably means slightly different things to different tribes; to parents, clinicians, research groups and activists. None of the tribes are homogeneous; there are many parents in the neurodiversity movement, for example, and within each there are different takes. The army of activists of autism, the tribes, has strongly influenced the definition of autism. The Autistic Self Advocacy Network (ASAN), for example, lobbied and advised the workgroup producing the fifth edition of the *Diagnostic and Statistical Manual of Mental Disorders* (DSM-5) and can point to tangible changes in the DSM criteria that their arguments solidified. An account of their actions is included in Kapp's *Exploring Diagnosis* collection.[1]

Probably the easiest way to answer the question *'what is autism?'* is to refer to widely used, standardised manuals such as the DSM, which at the time of writing is in its fifth edition (DSM-5),[26] most commonly used by clinicians in the USA, and increasingly in the UK, and the *International Classification of Diseases*, currently in its 11th iteration (ICD-11),[27] more commonly used in Europe. For the purposes of definition, let us consider autism to be what the DSM-5 says it is (Figure I.4).

The DSM positions autism as a characteristic of a person's development, yet acknowledges that social context affects how well a person with autism copes, and hopefully thrives. Both ICD-11 and DSM-5 list two core symptoms of autism: persistent deficits in social interaction and social communication and restricted, repetitive and inflexible patterns of behaviour and interests, including

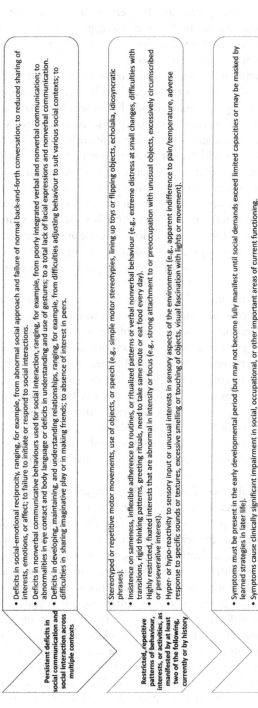

Persistent deficits in social communication and social interaction across multiple contexts

- Deficits in social-emotional reciprocity, ranging, for example, from abnormal social approach and failure of normal back-and-forth conversation; to reduced sharing of interests, emotions, or affect; to failure to initiate or respond to social interactions.
- Deficits in nonverbal communicative behaviours used for social interaction, ranging, for example, from poorly integrated verbal and nonverbal communication; to abnormalities in eye contact and body language or deficits in understanding and use of gestures; to a total lack of facial expressions and nonverbal communication.
- Deficits in developing, maintaining, and understanding relationships, ranging, for example, from difficulties adjusting behaviour to suit various social contexts; to difficulties in sharing imaginative play or in making friends; to absence of interest in peers.

Restricted, repetitive patterns of behaviour, interests, or activities, as manifested by at least two of the following, currently or by history

- Stereotyped or repetitive motor movements, use of objects, or speech (e.g., simple motor stereotypies, lining up toys or flipping objects, echolalia, idiosyncratic phrases).
- Insistence on sameness, inflexible adherence to routines, or ritualized patterns or verbal nonverbal behaviour (e.g., extreme distress at small changes, difficulties with transitions, rigid thinking patterns, greeting rituals, need to take same route or eat food every day).
- Highly restricted, fixated interests that are abnormal in intensity or focus (e.g., strong attachment to or preoccupation with unusual objects, excessively circumscribed or perseverative interest).
- Hyper- or hypo-reactivity to sensory input or unusual interests in sensory aspects of the environment (e.g., apparent indifference to pain/temperature, adverse response to specific sounds or textures, excessive smelling or touching of objects, visual fascination with lights or movement).

Other diagnostic criteria:

- Symptoms must be present in the early developmental period (but may not become fully manifest until social demands exceed limited capacities or may be masked by learned strategies in later life).
- Symptoms cause clinically significant impairment in social, occupational, or other important areas of current functioning.
- These disturbances are not better explained by intellectual disability (intellectual developmental disorder) or global developmental delay.

Figure I.4 Diagnostic criteria for autism in the fifth edition of the *Diagnostic and Statistical Manual of Mental Disorders* (DSM-5).

enhanced or diminished sensory perception. If a person shows these behaviours in different settings, a clinician would be able to give a diagnosis of autism. Because the behavioural traits show regardless of setting, they can better be attributed to atypical brain development than to social context.

The onset of autism typically occurs in early childhood but the ICD-11 notes that autism may not become obvious until later, which suggests the underlying way of functioning psychologically may already be present but that expression is less obvious because of the particular demands placed on children's roles at different ages. Of course, things may also develop differently given the exposures the child has as they grow up, which clearly affect these patterns of functioning. The point the criteria make is that autism can exist undetected in very young children. Both sets of diagnostic criteria describe behavioural traits as symptoms and look at the impact of said symptoms. According to the DSM-5, autism might 'limit or impair everyday functioning'. This emphasises the impact autism has on a person's ability to live a fulfilled and functioning life and paints autism as a condition that is primarily a set of psychological or behavioural traits, or an aspect of a person's character. Autism affects both other people and the person's ability to thrive.

Various psychological theories to explain autism have been put forward,[28] all of which have their supporters and detractors; no model seems comprehensive.[29] The merits of the various theories, many of which seem plausible, are not my focus. Autism might stem from sensory-processing differences,[30] including enhanced perceptual functioning,[31] weak central coherence,[32] lack of theory of mind,[33] an extreme male brain,[34] defects in the mirror neuron system[35] or the impairment of executive function,[36, 37] to name but a few. In a slow state of flux, its theories and diagnostic tools are somewhat circular or tautological. We study autism and derive a new psychological theory or diagnostic test. If this is how we then understand or measure autism, the new test or theory starts to shape the object that we subsequently understand autism to be. And this regulates who is in the category for study: a loop.

The presentations and abilities of people with autism are notoriously diverse.[38] Maija Nadesan goes so far as to suggest people diagnosed with autism today are united merely by being people who do not fit their social environment.[8] Those who qualify include people with severe intellectual disability and people with PhDs, those living independently and those in residential care, those with hyper-sensitivity and those with hypo-sensitivity, those who are remote and those who are over-attached, those who lack emotional response and those with anger problems, those who lack interest in others and those with apparently good (through feigned) social skills that allow them to 'blend in'. People diagnosed with autism might be completely non-verbal, be highly articulate or use idiosyncratic language; they might have repetitive motor movements, have special focused interests, lack imaginative play or the use of gestures or show great talent in acting, humour and the arts. Or any combination. Because of its heterogeneity, several attempts have been made to differentiate different forms by sub-typing.[39] Some researchers have suggested there are many 'autisms', with distinct genomic predispositions and perhaps separate cognitive profiles.[40] Responses to treatment also vary, which has led to calls for treatment and intervention studies to investigate outcomes for sub-types.[41–43]

Since the mid-1990s, the notion of a 'spectrum' has been central to autism research. The range and nature of the broader spectrum were brilliantly illustrated by Colin Steer and his colleagues,[44] who analysed more than 90 traits linked to autism in more than 13,000 children, both autistic and non-autistic. We adapted the idea in a later study based partly on the same dataset.[45] The results of our study, illustrated in Figure I.5, show autistic traits in a population-based sample of all children, regardless of whether they had a diagnosis. The *y*-axis represents the number of children in the study and the *x*-axis gives a score for each child on autistic-type traits. The results show autistic traits are reasonably normally distributed throughout the whole child population. Our measures also showed a 'tail' of more severe autism traits; unsurprisingly, many in this 'tail' received an autism diagnosis.

The spectrum that crosses the diagnosis boundary is known as the broad autism phenotype.[46] As Figure I.5 shows, almost all people have some measure of autism traits; some people have almost none, most people very few and some have many. It is only those with very severe traits who are diagnosed. A fairly arbitrary, culturally determined cut-off (Figure I.5) is used to separate people who have *diagnosable* autism from those who have less severe autistic traits. People with diagnosable autism near this boundary may not have a radically different profile from those beyond. It is a good jumping-off point for reviewing the evidence to show that autism-as-diagnosed is on the rise and address the reasons why.

As well as delineating who is eligible for diagnosis, the defining criteria have a huge impact on how people identify themselves, how others think of them, how

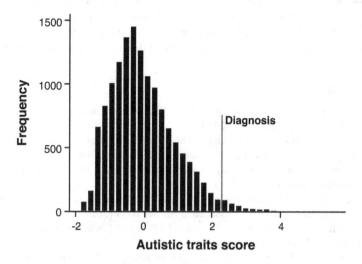

Figure I.5 Distribution of traits contributing to the autism spectrum.

they act and even perhaps how underlying neurological differences are expressed. Diagnoses describe biological differences but, once assigned, are used to interpret patients' differences and frame the differences within the diagnostic explanation or narrative. This book considers both how diagnostic classifications can transform the defined populations and, in turn, how these new populations can transform our understanding of the categories.

This book has taken more than a year to write and draws on ten years of research, particularly my work in epidemiology and qualitative research from my PhD studies, as well as later work from a study of time trends in neurodevelopmental diagnoses, funded by the Economic and Social Sciences Research Council (UK). The bulk of the work described here comes from qualitative research studies that were conducted as part of a Wellcome Trust-funded Investigator Award, *Exploring Diagnosis*. Broadly, the epidemiological work has been about autism diagnosis at a population level and the qualitative work about the meaning people make of diagnosis.

During these ten years, I have learned that understanding autism comes as much from the politics and processes of research as from the data that emerge from that research. This has allowed me to reflect on how our institutional practices – the way science is done – shape our work and consequently the stories that are told. Interacting with autistic adults and activists has equally shaped my work and I hope to describe how. As the book was finished during the 2020 coronavirus pandemic, I will be using the example of Covid-19 to punctuate a few of my points.

Does the world really need another social science book about autism? I hope to add something new by grounding the story in empirical studies and statistics, together with quotes and illustrated by graphics, an approach I hope will appeal to clinicians and visual thinkers like me. By looking at the identification of autism and 'risk of autism' through different stages of human life, I will consider the possibility that environmental changes and other modern-day phenomena have led to increased levels of autism and, I hope, move beyond the somewhat weary polarisation of autism as either neurodevelopmental difference or social construction.

References

1. Kapp, S. K. *Autistic Community and the Neurodiversity Movement: Stories from the Frontline* (Springer Singapore, 2020).
2. Haraway, D. Situated Knowledges: The Science Question in Feminism and the Privilege of Partial Perspective. *Fem. Stud.* **14**, 575–599 (1988).
3. Giddens, A. *Modernity and Self-Identity: Self and Society in the Late Modern Age* (Stanford University Press, 1991).
4. Russell, G. *et al.* Selection Bias on Intellectual Ability in Autism Research: A Cross-sectional Review and Meta-analysis. *Mol. Autism* **10**, 9 (2019).
5. Evans, B. *The Metamorphosis of Autism: A History of Child Development in Britain* (Manchester University Press, 2017).
6. Eyal, G., Hart, B., Onculer, E., Neta, O. & Rossi, N. *The Autism Matrix* (Polity, 2010).

7. Waltz, M. *Autism: A Social and Medical History* (Palgrave Macmillan, 2013).

8. Nadesan, M. *Constructing Autism: Unravelling the 'Truth' and Understanding the Social* (Routledge, 2005).

9. Feinstein, A. *A History of Autism: Conversations with the Pioneers* (Wiley-Blackwell, 2010).

10. Fombonne, E. Is There an Epidemic of Autism? *Pediatrics* **107**, 411–412 (2001).

11. Hacking, I. The Looping Effects of Human Kinds. In *Causal Cognition* (eds. Sperber, D., Premack, D. & Premack, A. J.) (Oxford University Press, 1996). doi:10.1093/acprof:oso/9780198524021.001.0001.

12. Watters, E. *Crazy Like Us: The Globalization of the American Psyche* (Free Press, 2010).

13. Rose, N. What is Diagnosis for? (2013). Royal College of Psychiatry. Conference on DSM-5 and the Future of Diagnosis. https://nikolasrose.com/wp-content/uploads/2013/07/Rose-2013-What-is-diagnosis-for-IoP-revised-July-2013.pdf

14. Silverman, C. Fieldwork on Another Planet: Social Science Perspectives on the Autism Spectrum. *BioSocieties* **3**, 325–341 (2008).

15. Silberman, S. *Neurotribes: The Legacy of Autism and How to Think Smarter About People Who Think Differently* (Allen & Unwin, 2015).

16. Ne'eman, A. The Future (and the Past) of Autism Advocacy, Or Why the ASA's Magazine, The Advocate, Wouldn't Publish This Piece. *Disabil. Stud. Q.* **30** (2010).

17. Silverman, C. *Understanding Autism: Parents, Doctors, and the History of a Disorder* (Princeton University Press, 2011).

18. Conrick, T. The Scientific and Basic Moral Reasons We Need an Autism Cure. *Age of Autism* (2013).

19. Baker, J. P. Mercury, Vaccines, and Autism. *Am. J. Public Health* **98**, 244–253 (2008).

20. Lister, T. *What's in a Label? An Exploration of How People Acquire the Label 'Autistic' in Adulthood and the Consequences of Doing So* (University of Exeter, 2020).

21. Dyck, E. & Russell, G. Challenging Psychiatric Classification: Healthy Autistic Diversity the Neurodiversity Movement. In *Mental Health in Historical Perspective: Healthy Minds in the Twentieth Century* (eds. Taylor, S. J. & Brumby, A.) (Palgrave MacMillan, 2020).

22. Broderick, A. A. & Ne'eman, A. Autism as Metaphor: Narrative and Counter-narrative. *Int. J. Incl. Educ.* **12**, 459–476 (2008).

23. Bowker, G. C. & Star, S. L. *Sorting Things Out: Classification and Its Consequences* (The MIT Press, 2000).

24. Leigh Star, S. This is Not a Boundary Object: Reflections on the Origin of a Concept. *Sci. Technol. Hum. Values* **35**, 601–617 (2010).

25. Aronowitz, R. A. When do Symptoms Become a Disease? *Ann. Intern. Med.* **134**, 803–808 (2001).

26. American Psychiatric Association & DSM-5 Task Force. *Diagnostic and Statistical Manual of Mental Disorders: DSM-5* (American Psychiatric Association, 2013).

27. WHO. *International Classification of Diseases, 11th Revision (ICD-11)* (WHO, 2018). www.who.int/classifications/icd/en/.

28. Levy, F. Theories of Autism. *Aust. N. Z. J. Psychiatry* **41**, 859–868 (2007).

29. Happé, F. G. Current Psychological Theories of Autism: The 'Theory of Mind' Account and Rival Theories. *J. Child Psychol. Psychiatry* **35**, 215–229 (1994).

30. Gallagher, S. & Varga, S. Conceptual Issues in Autism Spectrum Disorders. *Curr. Opin. Psychiatry* **28**, 127–132 (2015).

31. Mottron, L., Dawson, M., Soulières, I., Hubert, B. & Burack, J. Enhanced Perceptual Functioning in Autism: An Update, and Eight Principles of Autistic Perception. *J. Autism Dev. Disord.* **36**, 27–43 (2006).

32. Happé, F. & Frith, U. The Weak Coherence Account: Detail-focused Cognitive Style in Autism Spectrum Disorders. *J. Autism Dev. Disord.* **36**, 5–25 (2006).
33. Baron-Cohen, S., Leslie, A. M. & Frith, U. Does the Autistic Child Have a 'Theory of Mind'? *Cognition* **21**, 37–46 (1985).
34. Baron-Cohen, S. The Extreme Male Brain Theory of Autism. *Trends Cogn. Sci.* **6**, 248–254 (2002).
35. Iacoboni, M. & Dapretto, M. The Mirror Neuron System and the Consequences of its Dysfunction. *Nat. Rev. Neurosci.* **7**, 942–951 (2006).
36. Craig, F. *et al.* A Review of Executive Function Deficits in Autism Spectrum Disorder and Attention-deficit/Hyperactivity Disorder. *Neuropsychiatr. Dis. Treat.* **12**, 1191–1202 (2016).
37. Russell, J., Jarrold, C. & Henry, L. Working Memory in Children with Autism and with Moderate Learning Difficulties. *J. Child Psychol. Psychiatry* **37**, 673–686 (2006).
38. Baird, G., Cass, H. & Slonims, V. Diagnosis of Autism. *BMJ* **327**, 488–493 (2003).
39. Bölte, S. Is Autism Curable? *Dev. Med. Child Neurol.* **56**, 927–931 (2014).
40. Coleman, M. & Gillberg, C. *The Autisms* (Oxford University Press, USA, 2012).
41. Loth, E., Murphy, D. G. & Spooren, W. Defining Precision Medicine Approaches to Autism Spectrum Disorders: Concepts and Challenges. *Front. Psychiatry* **7** (2016).
42. Persico, A. M. & Napolioni, V. Autism Genetics. *Behav. Brain Res.* 95–112 (2013).
43. Warren, Z. *et al.* A Systematic Review of Early Intensive Intervention for Autism Spectrum Disorders. *Pediatrics* **127**, e1303–e1311 (2011).
44. Steer, C. D., Golding, J. & Bolton, P. F. Traits Contributing to the Autistic Spectrum. *PLoS One* **5**, e12633 (2010).
45. Russell, G., Collishaw, S., Golding, J., Kelly, S. E. & Ford, T. Changes in Diagnosis Rates and Behavioural Traits of Autism Spectrum Disorders Over Time. *BJPsych Open* **1**(2), 110–115 (2015) doi:10.1192/bjpo.bp.115.000976.
46. Piven, J. The Broad Autism Phenotype: A Complementary Strategy for Molecular Genetic Studies of Autism. *Am. J. Med. Genet.* **105**, 34–35 (2001).

1   Establishing the trend

The rising use of the autism diagnosis

My academic research has involved analysing data, both quantitative (numbers) and qualitative (texts or conversations). In epidemiological studies, I have examined the numbers of children with autism diagnoses and their change over time.[1,2] Many other researchers have covered similar ground, measuring autism in different ways, sometimes using a research diagnosis, sometimes clinical reports or parental reports of diagnosis.[3-8] The graphs in this chapter show some of the published data on autism time trends in Europe and the USA. To establish the trends, I have used multiple datasets from many sources. Rather than reading as monotonous, I hope this will harness the power of repetition.

Prevalence is the number of people in a population who have a condition, relative to the total population, typically shown as a percentage. Each data point in Figure 1.1–1.5 represent the estimated percentage of children who had autism at that time. Figure 1.1 shows the time trend in prevalence estimates from the 1970s into the 2000s; the earlier data (up to 2011) originate from an article in *Nature* ('The prevalence puzzle'[9]) and the later data from the Centers for Disease Control and Prevention (CDC) in the USA.[10]

The earliest estimates hark back to the first epidemiological studies of autism that were carried out in the UK by Victor Lotter and his team in 1966[11] and in the USA by Darold Treffert, published four years later.[12] Lotter estimated about one in 2,500 children had autism and the first study by Treffert estimated that fewer than one child in every 10,000 had autism. At that time, autism was considered an extremely rare condition and was almost always associated with intellectual disability.

Figure 1.1 gives an overall, and quite compelling, impression of an exponential increase in the use of the label of autism. But it is debatable how directly comparable the early data in Figure 1.1 are with the later data, as studies use different methods to establish exactly who has autism, as well as having a wide geographic spread.

To get over some the limitations of Figure 1.1's geographical and methodological disjointedness, it is worth looking at other datasets. The data in Figure 1.2, which are publicly available, were all taken from CDC data. Since 2000, this

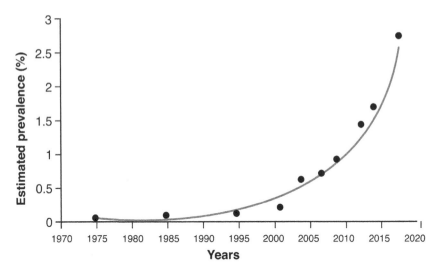

Figure 1.1 Post-1970 time trend in estimated prevalence of autism.

American centre has repeatedly used the same methods to measure how many children (from an enormous sample of more than 300,000) have autism.[10] The data, of children of eight years old, are recorded in 11 sites around the USA, a process repeated every few years. In this huge study, researchers obtain children's evaluation records from data sources in the community. Experienced clinicians review these records to determine whether the behaviours described are consistent with the diagnostic criteria for autism. Children with a documented autism diagnosis are also included in their case definition. The period it covers, 2000–2012, therefore uses comparable methodology and sampling methods to create the time trend and so gets round some of the problems of compatibility. Because methods of case ascertainment remained more or less stable, the numbers through time are more directly equivalent. Figure 1.2 illustrates how the estimated prevalence of autism has risen year on year. In 2014, there was a 15% increase from two years before (2012), when 1.7% of children reportedly had autism, and a 150% increase since 2000. The last estimate, reported in 2014, included in Figure 1.2, is that by the age of eight 1.68% of children have autism, which translates to one in every 59 children. The linear time trend provides the best fit, according to some *post hoc* work done by our PhD student, Rhianna White.

Another dataset, plotted in Figure 1.3, is taken from the US National Health Interview Survey (NHIS). These results were published in 2018 in a letter in the *Journal of the American Medical Association* (*JAMA*) and estimated the prevalence of autism in 2016 at 2.7%.[13] Unlike the CDC study, this is a nationally representative sample, meaning one in every 37 American children is reported to have identified autism in 2016. The estimates from the NHIS are obtained in telephone interviews with parents of children and adolescents. The latest sample

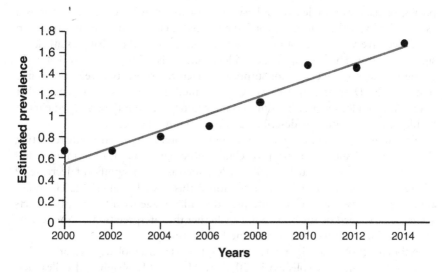

Figure 1.2 Twenty-first-century time trend from prevalence estimates.

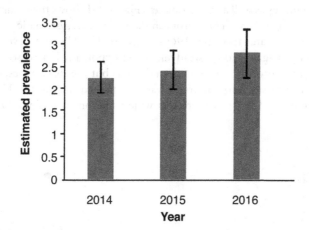

Figure 1.3 National Health Interview Survey data.

comprised around 30,000 parents of children between the ages of three and 17. They were asked: 'has a doctor or health professional ever told you that [your child] has autism, Asperger's disorder, pervasive developmental disorder or autism spectrum disorder?' These are all conditions on the autism spectrum – forms of autism as we know it today.

The NHIS data also have their limitations. Arguably, the question's phrasing has led to an over-estimate of the number of children identified as having a diagnosis of autism. Parents could interpret 'health professional' to mean a number of professionals, for example a school psychologist who may have mentioned autism as a possibility, without it being confirmed. Nevertheless, using the same question in consecutive years, the estimates show a consistent, although not statistically significant, rise. The overlapping confidence intervals shown in Figure 1.3, indicating non-significance, are not surprising, given the short, two-year, timeframe under study. Despite this, the work was framed in the press as evidence that autism was stable, a somewhat dubious interpretation; from the observed data, it would more accurately be described as a non-significant rise.

This draws our attention to language and interpretation. In an article reporting the reducing chances of autism for children receiving the measles, mumps and rubella (MMR) vaccine, such an effect is described as 'a non-significant decrease'.[14] There is no link between MMR and autism; this is well established. The point is rather that how the data are interpreted and language used to describe effects seems to be shaped by the body politic: whether the interpretation fits the acceptable scientific narrative. This is a theme I will return to.

A fourth set of data (Figures 1.4 and 1.5) harks from a global systematic review of autism prevalence published in 2012 by Mayada Elsabbagh and colleagues. They drew on more than 25 epidemiological studies that estimated autism prevalence in different locations around the world,[15] using a variety of methods to identify autism cases. The authors published prevalence estimates from 11 European countries as well as US estimates (Figure 1.4 shows their European and Figure 1.5 their US data). The European data from this systematic review show steadily rising estimates from the 1960s to 2010. The US data cover the trend over 40 years and again show a steady increase. Exponential increases are significant in both the European and American datasets but the shallow best-fit line for the European data suggests the trend was less marked than in the USA during the early 2000s, and in both there was wide variation by region. The authors

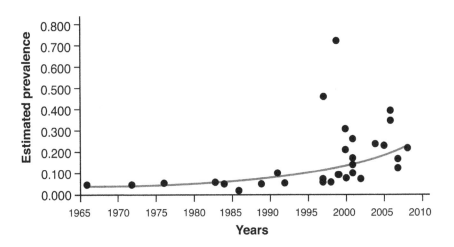

Figure 1.4 Prevalence estimates of autism in European countries.

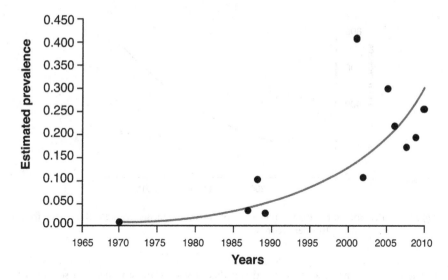

Figure 1.5 Prevalence estimates in the USA.

conclude that their review provides clear evidence of increasing estimates over time in both continents. The exponential trend is significant in both datasets but not as good a fit to the data as other figures seen here.

These data suffer from the same limitations as the data in Figure 1.1, in that data points on the graphs use different methods of case ascertainment and each is from a different place. In Europe, in particular, there is wide variation in geography, culture and the methods used to ascertain autism. On the other hand, these data are valuable because they draw on many studies which were sampled in a systematic, and therefore replicable, way.

This brief review provides pretty compelling evidence for the rise of autism internationally, although the data are somewhat dated, as there is a time lag between gathering and publication. I am writing from the UK, so what of the UK situation?

We examined the increase in incidence of autism diagnosis as recorded by family doctors, known as general practitioners (GPs) in England.[1] GPs report on their patients using diagnostic codes, providing an enormous population-based sample of more than nine million people. We examined incidence – in other words, new recordings – of cases of autism (Figure 1.6 shows the best fit line of the index number: that is, starting at 100% in 1998, which was the baseline year, and plotting the increase in percentage relative to 100% at each year. So 120% represents 20% increase in recorded cases). Again, we found the exponential trend was the best fit to describe the time trend over a 20-year period – an exponential trend in new cases, not a cumulative prevalence estimate which would have shown an even steeper trend. Year on year there have been more new cases of autism recorded than in the previous year, over the 20-year timeframe. Granted, the GP dataset is

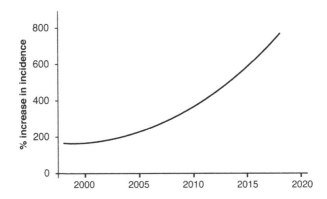

Figure 1.6 Percentage increase in incidence of autism diagnosis from 1998 to 2018 from general practitioner records.

not ideal for studying autism, as autism diagnoses are mostly made in secondary care diagnostic assessment services, which accept school, public health nursing and sometimes self- or parent-referrals, as well as referrals by GPs. This means diagnoses may not always be sent back to GPs from secondary care. Additionally, some GPs are better at recording than others and their diligence may have increased with time. The figure shows the rate of growth in cases recorded not absolute prevalence of autism increasing. Nevertheless, an overall increase in incidence of diagnosis of autism is consistent with other reports and datasets in the USA and Europe.

In 2013, we published data from the UK Millennium Cohort Study (MCS) which covers more than 19,000 British children.[16] Our estimates from these data suggested that at seven or eight years old, 1.7% of children had been identified with autism. Like the NHIS studies, this was based on parents' reports of diagnosis. In our MCS study and the GP dataset we were concerned not with the absolute prevalence of autism, but of autism diagnosis as our object of study; on rates of recognition of autism, rather than on the number of children with high levels of behavioural traits characteristic of autism with or without recognition. The MCS is a longitudinal study, tracking children through time, with some drop-out of participants as time passes (known by epidemiologists as attrition), which sometimes skews results. Having said that, the survey provides data weightings designed to estimate findings that are generalisable to the UK (that is, representative of the national picture).

In 2018, we re-estimated the percentage of children in the UK with autism using MCS data from when they were 14, an update from eight years old. The new number gave us pause for thought. We found a prevalence of 3.07% (95% confidence interval (CI) 2.64–3.57) – higher than we had ever seen reported. If we simply reported what the data told us, we were concerned our estimate might be misinterpreted, as it seemed exceptionally high – too large an increase from eight years old. By misinterpreted I mean that people might read that autism rates had jumped, rather than that recognition (and possibly parental reporting) of autism had jumped. Although the increase might partly be due to more children being diagnosed after eight and before 14 years old, the increase was too marked to explain away completely and we decided not to publish our report. In a sense, we self-censored our findings; an example of one small mechanism of shaping what comes to be published. I will delve into the context of why we made this choice later.

Looking for an absolute prevalence is perhaps misguided. As discussed in the introduction, autistic traits are a normally distributed set of multi-dimensional traits in the broad population;[17] who qualifies as having autism is shaped by where an arbitrary cut-off for severity is imposed. There is no 'true' prevalence; the severity of autism that qualifies as 'having autism' has clearly changed over time. No magic number can tell us how many people have autism; it all depends where the inclusion criteria, the boundaries, are drawn. Instead, prevalence estimates tell us about how we conceive autism, at how good we are at identifying it in a given place and a given era.

The flawed NHIS question means neither NHIS nor the MCS employs the best methods for estimating the prevalence of autism. Each source of data can be criticised; each has its strengths and limitations. In particular, there is often a trade-off in epidemiology between collecting data from huge samples on a national scale and those studies with smaller, more focused samples in which the methods of case ascertainment can be addressed more thoroughly. Smaller samples often have the capacity to use more comprehensive measures of autism, the so-called gold-standard approach, in which clinical raters confirm a diagnosis. But such methods may not be nationally representative, so estimates may not be generalisable to the population of a whole nation, for example.

Epidemiology is quite a contested science and prevalence estimates are generated in quite different ways. Global systematic reviews of prevalence often depend on the underlying assumption that there is an identifiable fixed psychiatric construct with a primarily biological/genetic aetiology; a universality. Conditions should, in theory, be stable in their prevalence everywhere. Therefore, global prevalence studies of autism (and attention deficit hyperactivity disorder (ADHD), and other medical diagnoses) have emphasised interpretations that show a steadiness of rates across borders, another mechanism of shaping understandings of categories as universal. Variations in rates globally (which are wide) are dismissed as likely to be artefacts of measurement.

Ironically, estimates that try to establish the prevalence of condition X are themselves used to reify conditions as having a fixed prevalence. One example is the estimate of global prevalence of ADHD; that around 5% of children have ADHD.[18] Because this figure was widely published and disseminated, it has become a baseline against which to assess under- or over-diagnosis. For example, UK ADHD prevalence estimates are lower, hovering around 3%.[19] This lower rate than the global estimate is attributed in the psychiatric literature to use of more stringent *International Classification of Diseases* (ICD) criteria in the UK. Yet I have heard speakers at ADHD conferences claim the UK discrepancy with the global estimate shows that ADHD is under-diagnosed in the UK. This makes little sense: if you set a boundary of severity of ADHD at 5%, it means the 5% of the population that is most hyperactive and inattentive qualifies for diagnosis. If the boundary were 2%, the top 2% would have ADHD and if set at 10%, then 10%, and so on.[20] Although neurological differences are real, the borders of neurodevelopmental categories are artefactual. There is no one 'correct' situation or practice.

The focus of this book is not the absolute prevalence of autism in any given population but rather the time trend; why autism, as diagnosed in the clinic, by researchers, or by other people, is on the rise. *Taken together*, the figures and data illustrate with confidence that the time trend in autism diagnosis and identification is upward. *All* the datasets give a similar picture, despite their various limits, fluctuations and problems, so we can say with some certainty that more children are being classified with autism. Taken overall, all the sources of evidence seem to point to one conclusion: there is a consistent rise in the *use and application* of the label and category of autism over time. Autism diagnosis has been on the rise.

Different interpretations

My question is *why* more children are identified with autism today than before. To recap, most epidemiologists, clinicians and researchers have argued the rise is solely an *artefact* of changing diagnostic practice, the expanding boundaries of the diagnostic category of autism and other cultural changes.[21, 22] They contend that the observed change is not due to more people having autism; we simply apply the label more frequently. In this view, an autism diagnosis is a categorical class, whose boundaries are constructed by human agency and shifts in its construction are solely responsible for the observed rise. Nobody denies artefactual changes have led to a massive increase in the use of the diagnosis but other groups, mostly parent activists and some notable clinicians, have argued the rise may also be attributable to an actual increase in the proportion of children who display traits characteristic of autism. For this group, the rise is likely to be partially *real*; there really are more children with autism today than ever before.

On both sides of the argument the more extreme proponents hold entrenched positions. Some parent advocates vociferously declare there is an autism 'epidemic' and produce evidence they cite as a fact. In authoritative tones, respected scientists declare autism rates are stable and produce evidence to attest this. Many researchers in the autism field fall between these two camps; they admit that both arguments are plausible, that the trend is clearly artefactual but there is possibly also a 'true' component. The debate as to whether autism is *really* on the rise remains unresolved, as acknowledged by the fifth edition of the *Diagnostic and Statistical Manual of Mental Disorders* (DSM-5):

> *It remains unclear whether higher rates reflect an expansion of the diagnostic criteria of DSM-IV to include sub-threshold cases, increased awareness,*

differences in study methodology or a true increase in the frequency of autism spectrum disorder.[23]

In their global review, Elsabbagh and colleagues[15] conclude that, while it is clear that prevalence estimates have increased over time, the findings most probably represent a broadening of the diagnostic concept, a diagnostic switching from other developmental disabilities to autism, service availability and awareness of autism in both the lay and professional public; that is, artefactual shifts. This is pretty typical of the constructivist interpretation of most epidemiologists and academic researchers: the rise in autism can be attributed to changes in the way autism is measured, the broadening of the category and improved identification as clinicians become more knowledgeable about autism and parents are more forthcoming about their children's differences and difficulties. Artefactual shifts such as these highlight the constructed nature not perhaps of the category of neurodevelopmental difference but of the human agency in deciding where the boundaries of the category lie and how they are defined and measured.

No one can seriously doubt that artefactual shifts have accounted for a huge rise in cases. What is striking in the conclusions of the aforementioned authors[15] is that, although they declare their findings show the marked rise and explain it in terms of the three points made above, they make no mention of the obvious fourth possible explanation: *that there really are more children with autism today than previously*. Put another way, there is a higher proportion of children and adults displaying traits characteristic of autism (and consequently also a higher proportion with identified autism) in more recent generations than can be accounted for by artefactual shifts alone. This would mean there has been a true increase in prevalence of autism world-wide.

Biopolitics of autism

The reason for silence, and why we were nervous to publish our MCS finding, may be because the suggestion of any real increase is so inflammatory. Most probably, if there is truly a rise in autism cases it is attributable to a new environmental or social risk factor.

One 'tribe' was at the centre of what has been described as the biggest scandal in public health in the last three decades.[24] The story of how autism was linked to the MMR vaccine by the notorious (and now retracted) scientific paper by Andrew Wakefield and colleagues, and how this paper subsequently became a rallying call for anti-vaccine parent activists, sends shivers down the spines of public health experts. Writing in the *British Medical Journal*, David Oliver[24] claims every scientific paper that could be cast as being in support of the anti-vaccine cause (whatever its quality) and every commentator sympathetic to the anti-vaccine cause (expert or not) is selectively harvested and cited by anti-vaccine activists.

Despite many studies showing there is no link between autism and vaccines,[25] including an enormous Danish study refuting a link to MMR[26] and a systematic review,[27] there are still many anti-vaccine activists and many parents loath to vaccinate their children. In 2018, the UK rates of vaccination against MMR in under-10s fell for the sixth consecutive year. Between 2010 and 2017 an estimated half a million children missed their MMR vaccination. [24] Public health bodies have issued dire warnings about the rise of measles due to an 'epidemic' of unvaccinated children.

Anti-vaccine activists are a committed bunch of people, who have been hugely successful in disrupting the roll-out of vaccines. In the USA, active groups of parents, known as the 'Mercury Moms', have focused on concern about the mercury-based preservative thimerosal which, although it has now been eliminated from routine childhood vaccines, is present in many vaccines in the USA. Parent vaccine activists mobilised around autism have been vociferous in arguing their position in both Europe and the USA, as evidenced by the on-going newsletter *The Age of Autism*, which calls itself the 'Daily Web Newspaper of the Autism Epidemic'. The lack of uptake of vaccines has prompted an outbreak of measles in the UK and was termed 'a public health timebomb' by the head of National Health England, who also called for a ban on social media sites of anti-vaccination propaganda, such as anti-vax endorsement from celebrities such as Jim Carrey and Robert de Niro.[28]

In this loaded bio-political climate, it is not surprising there is nervousness in the scientific establishment about how reports of increasing rates of autism will be received. The political environment also plays a role in both the muted interpretation of results and the decision not to publish studies. The US NHIS report in *JAMA* (the time trend shown in Figure 1.3) is a good example. The report was covered by multiple media platforms, including *CBS News, Fox News, Time* and *Scientific American*. To me, the data in Figure 1.3 look like a small snapshot of the larger trend: that year on year there is a rise in the use of autism as a diagnostic label. However, in media coverage, it was reported as evidence to show that autism was stable. 'US autism rates appear to be stabilising' declared CBS, whilst *Scientific American* led with 'The prevalence of autism in the US appears to be steady'.

When I asked a senior professor involved in the US NHIS study why the trend had been reported as stable, she expressed the authors' concern that the study would backfire; in other words (the wrong) people might misinterpret the results. The *'wrong people'* – meaning anti-vax activists – might use the study as further ammunition to support claims that there is a real rise in the levels and preponderance of autism, one triggered by an environmental risk. Anti-vax activists, on the other hand, would argue the 'acceptable' autism narratives are those the scientific establishment are telling and what is heard is determined by power relations, that is, they have to be active and take extreme measures to get their voices heard, compared to the scientific establishment. Similarly, despite simply reporting the data in front of us, we were worried about publishing the high estimate from the MCS data, because ours was so much higher than previous estimates.

Omitting to mention of the chance of a 'real' rise in the systematic review, countless media articles arguing the rates of autism are stable, the hesitancy to publish on UK increases – these are mechanisms that shape the story of suppression and selective interpretation. Perhaps not a conscious suppression but one born of the current climate set by anti-vaccine activism and the declarations of national public health institutions. When reading papers, it is important to remind ourselves from which discipline the conclusions originate and against what context the position is taken and the conclusion is drawn.

Looking across all the material, including some of our own (more on this later), it seems suggesting that the rise of autism could in any sense be 'real' is strongly discouraged by establishment science, perhaps for understandable reasons. The global systematic review's caution in naming a real rise as a possibility and the *JAMA* paper's press coverage that autism rates are stable suggest skewing and shaping of what can and can't be published. Is the institutional pressure to only publish the 'correct' medical narrative around autism diagnosis helpful?

The more established narrative is that:

1. There is no objective rise in the prevalence of autism.
2. It only seems that there is because:
   (a) changing diagnostic thresholds and other artefactual issues inflate figures, thereby creating a misperception of increased prevalence; nevertheless, reduced thresholds remain socially and culturally desirable because people who have a recognised disability can get better support.
   (b) scholarly studies claiming that there is a real increase are methodologically flawed.
   (c) non-scholarly anecdotal reports for causes of a real rise are misperceptions (the sub-text is they are made by unhinged people without tangible expertise).

My argument is that there needs to be methodological rigour; this is a disciplinary given. Despite this, the data in this chapter, taken together, demonstrate significant shifts over time that are, at the very least, thought provoking. Completely denying the possibility that autism really is more prevalent is difficult to justify. The rise in autism is a case in which selective interpretation of data, selective publication and the political context in which scientific institutions sit have shaped scientific discourse.

References

1. Russell, G. *et al.* Time Trends in Autism Diagnosis Over 20 Years: A UK Population-based Cohort Study (in development).
2. Russell, G., Collishaw, S., Golding, J., Kelly, S. E. & Ford, T. Changes in Diagnosis Rates and Behavioural Traits of Autism Spectrum Disorders Over Time. *BJPsych Open* 1(2), 110–115 (2015). doi:10.1192/bjpo.bp.115.000976.

3. Lundström, S., Reichenberg, A., Anckarsäter, H., Lichtenstein, P. & Gillberg, C. Autism Phenotype Versus Registered Diagnosis in Swedish Children: Prevalence Trends Over 10 years in General Population Samples. *BMJ* **350** (2015).

4. Parner, E. T., Schendel, D. E. & Thorsen, P. Autism Prevalence Trends Over Time in Denmark: Changes in Prevalence and Age at Diagnosis. *Arch. Pediatr. Adolesc. Med.* **162**, 1150–1156 (2008).

5. Keyes, K. M. *et al.* Cohort Effects Explain the Increase in Autism Diagnosis Among Children Born from 1992 to 2003 in California. *Int. J. Epidemiol.* **41**, 495–503 (2012).

6. Smeeth, L. *et al.* Rate of First Recorded Diagnosis of Autism and Other Pervasive Developmental Disorders in United Kingdom General Practice, 1988 to 2001. *BMC Med.* **2**, 39 (2004).

7. Maenner, M. J. & Durkin, M. S. Trends in the Prevalence of Autism on the Basis of Special Education Data. *Pediatrics* **126**, e1018–e1025 (2010).

8. Boyle, C. A. *et al.* Trends in the Prevalence of Developmental Disabilities in US Children, 1997–2008. *Pediatrics* **127**, 1034–1042 (2011).

9. Weintraub, K. The Prevalence Puzzle: Autism Counts. *Nat. News* **479**, 22–24 (2011).

10. Centers for Disease Control and Prevention. *Data and Statistics on Autism Spectrum Disorder.* Autism Spectrum Disorder (ASD). www.cdc.gov/ncbddd/autism/data. html (2019).

11. Lotter, V. Epidemiology of Autistic Conditions in Young Children. *Soc. Psychiatry* **1**, 124–135 (1966).

12. Treffert, D. A. Epidemiology of Infantile Autism. *Arch. Gen. Psychiatry* **22**, 431–438 (1970).

13. Xu, G., Strathearn, L., Liu, B. & Bao, W. Prevalence of Autism Spectrum Disorder Among US Children and Adolescents, 2014–2016. *JAMA* **319**, 81–82 (2018).

14. Modabbernia, A., Velthorst, E. & Reichenberg, A. Environmental Risk Factors for Autism: An Evidence-based Review of Systematic Reviews and Meta-analyses. *Mol. Autism* **8**, 13 (2017).

15. Elsabbagh, M. *et al.* Global Prevalence of Autism and Other Pervasive Developmental Disorders. *Autism Res.* **5**, 160–179 (2012).

16. Russell, G., Rodgers, L. R., Ukoumunne, O. C. & Ford, T. Prevalence of Parent-Reported ASD and ADHD in the UK: Findings from the Millennium Cohort Study. *J. Autism Dev. Disord.* 1–10 (2013) doi:10.1007/s10803-013-1849-0.

17. Steer, C. D., Golding, J. & Bolton, P. F. Traits Contributing to the Autistic Spectrum. *PLoS One* **5**, e12633 (2010).

18. Polanczyk, G. V., Salum, G. A., Sugaya, L. S., Caye, A. & Rohde, L. A. Annual Research Review: A Meta-analysis of the Worldwide Prevalence of Mental Disorders in Children and Adolescents. *J. Child Psychol. Psychiatry* **56**, 345–365 (2015).

19. Ford, T., Goodman, R. & Meltzer, H. The British Child and Adolescent Mental Health Survey 1999: The Prevalence of DSM-IV Disorders. *J. Am. Acad. Child Adolesc. Psychiatry* **42**, 1203–1211 (2003).

20. Russell, G. & Ford, T. The Costs and Benefits of Diagnosis of ADHD: Commentary on Holden et al. *Child Adolesc. Psychiatry Ment. Health* **8**, 7 (2014).

21. Gernsbacher, M. A., Dawson, M. & Hill Goldsmith, H. Three Reasons Not to Believe in an Autism Epidemic. *Curr. Dir. Psychol. Sci.* **14**, 55–58 (2005).

22. Fombonne, E. Is There an Epidemic of Autism? *Pediatrics* **107**, 411–412 (2001).

23. American Psychiatric Association & DSM-5 Task Force. *Diagnostic and Statistical Manual of Mental Disorders: DSM-5* (American Psychiatric Association, 2013).

24. Oliver, D. David Oliver: Vaccination Sceptics are Immune to Debate. *BMJ* **365**, 12244 (2019).

25. Doja, A. & Roberts, W. Immunizations and Autism: A Review of the Literature. *Can. J. Neurol. Sci. J. Can. Sci. Neurol.* **33**, 341–346 (2006).

26. Hviid, A., Hansen, J. V., Frisch, M. & Melbye, M. Measles, Mumps, Rubella Vaccination and Autism: A Nationwide Cohort Study. *Ann. Intern. Med.* **170**, 513 (2019).

27. Taylor, L. E., Swerdfeger, A. L. & Eslick, G. D. Vaccines are not Associated with Autism: An Evidence-based Meta-analysis of Case-control and Cohort Studies. *Vaccine* **32**, 3623–3629 (2014).

28. Bodkin, H. Measles: Half a Million UK Children Unvaccinated Amid Fears of 'Public Health Timebomb'. *The Telegraph* 25 April (2019).

Part I

'Artefactual'

2   Babies and infants

Age of identification

'The earlier intervention can begin, the better the outcome.'[1]

Data from both the USA (e.g. California[2]) and Europe (e.g. Denmark[3]), show that the average and median ages at which childhood autism diagnoses are made are steadily dropping. However, there are some subtleties in the pattern; for example, our analysis[4] suggested that in England the average age of diagnosis for the youngest children (0–2 years) went up marginally between 1998 and 2018, perhaps because of increased demand for diagnoses and long waiting times.

Claims for identification of pre-symptomatic predictors of autism are now being made for very young babies.[5, 6] Using brain imaging, one group has noted autism-specific 'features' in six-month-old babies,[7] while another, which received world-wide media attention, used eye-tracking technology to identify subtle differences in the way affected babies responded to visual prompts:[8] 'Autism can be identified in babies as young as two months, early research suggests'.[9] Studies such as these, and others, are used to define infants 'at risk' of autism. To be 'at risk' is to be in danger of falling outside the statistical norm – a state requiring expert advice, intervention, parental regulation and surveillance.

The narrative of earlier-is-better (EIB) transcends autism to pervade child psychiatry, education and infant development and beyond: dementia, diabetes and hypertension spring to mind as examples of ways in which medicine has extended its jurisdiction.[10] Identifying potential early signs and signals of autism makes earlier diagnosis, detection and intervention possible. However, although the evidence base is regularly reviewed, the evidence that earlier intervention results in more successful outcomes for the child is poor.[11, 12] A recent UK review of evidence on screening infants for autism, conducted in 2011, concluded:

- Diagnoses of very young children may not be stable.
- Current screening tools are insufficiently sensitive and may not be accepted by a significant proportion of parents.
- The outcomes of interventions are variable.
- It is not known if short-term improvements continue in the long term.[13]

Baby-sibs

The collection of studies known as 'baby-sibs' research gives 'at-risk' status to new-born and unborn children who have siblings with autism.[14] At-risk status is given because autism is heritable and geneticised.[15–18] Sharing a genomic profile with autistic siblings, that is, being a sibling of someone with autism, therefore puts you at risk of autism. Estimates of the extent of familial heritability over 40 years ago were that around 90% of variance in autistic traits is attributable to inherited factors,[19] whereas today around 50% of variance is attributed to inherited factors.[20]

These two types of identification of the youngest children (an autism diagnosis in babyhood and the 'at-risk' status given to babies and unborn children) are related but distinct processes. Earlier autism diagnosis has consistently been associated with more severe autism and more severe impairment.[21–26] In childhood studies, the factors associated with an earlier diagnosis include greater language delay, need for a greater degree of support, more cognitive and intellectual disability, greater parental concern, an autism (as opposed to Asperger's) diagnosis and the severity of autistic beahviours.[21–26] The picture is one in which more severe autism is more obvious, therefore is picked up earlier in a child's life. Put simply, babies with more extreme neurodevelopmental difference are, and were before 1990, easier to spot.

A raft of EIB studies tells the story of how the earlier a child can be recognised, the more effective early intervention is, and so it must be brought into place.[27–30] The longer diagnosis is delayed, the greater the chances of missing a critical developmental period.[22] Once this window is missed, brain plasticity is lost and interventions may be ineffective.

At-risk babies (such as baby siblings, through their shared inheritance of a genetic predisposition) may be anywhere in the broad autism phenotype, which includes sub-clinical (milder) levels of autistic traits.[31] Baby-sibs studies look for early indicators of autism but necessarily include children who go on to develop milder, and in some cases, few or zero, autistic traits. Many but not all, baby-sibs studies follow up on later autism diagnosis.

Precursor signs of autism in infants, which have been deduced from baby-sibs and retrospective studies, can be loosely divided into behavioural signs, genetic predisposition and neurological differences. *Behaviours* include types of movements or lack of motor skills, imitation impairments, lack of physical exploration of objects in the environment with less object manipulation[32] and lack of joint attention. Many studies identify abnormal movement as a precursor, including gross motor, fine motor and postural control[28, 33–36] and babies' head lag.[37]

The larger catchment of 'at risk' of, as opposed to diagnosed with, autism presumably results in some studies widening the net of potential early signs of autism gleaned from siblings' behaviours and abilities. An aspect that is not often dwelt on is that a researcher denoting a baby sibling as 'at risk' surely makes an autism diagnosis more likely, not only through relatedness but also if parents see their baby as being in a proto-autism group. This, one would assume, will increase the likelihood of referral to a clinic and, once in the clinic, the interpretation of behaviour as autism. At the same time, by defining new signs of precursor autism using behaviours in the 'at-risk' group, all 'at-risk' babies' behaviours start to be understood as signalling autism. It seems circular: what counts as a specific 'signifier' of autism, most often motor difficulties, becomes connected to identification of autism in the group from whom the 'signifier' was determined.

Earlier diagnosis and risk

As well as identifying early indicators, autism studies have early diagnosis of autism as a core objective.[38] EIB is most commonly operationalised in intervention research. The assumption is that there is a fixed disorder that is present from birth, can be correctly identified soon after birth and which intervention will ameliorate. Advocacy, funding and charity organisations also strongly promote earlier diagnosis; for example, Autistica's report, *One in a Hundred*, emphasises the importance of diagnosis at the youngest possible age.[39] This report is typical of policy guidelines in higher-income countries but the rhetoric of early diagnosis is also visible in narratives aimed at broader publics. In the USA, five million coffee cups were released by Starbucks in a campaign aimed at raising the profile of autism, put together by the founder of the charity *Autism Speaks* (Figure 2.1).

In an inspired analysis, Anne McGuire argued the Coffee Cup casts the non-normatively developing child as non-valuable and perhaps even non-viable in a market-driven economy (of Starbucks).[40] Certainly, this widely distributed declaration contributed to the cultural recognition of autism as a threat, something to be dreaded and something to be identified (by parents' surveillance) as early as possible so that it can be fixed. And the younger the better. It also invokes a moral obligation for parents to monitor their children, if they wish to qualify as good parents.

The Coffee Cup uses non-gender-specific language. Despite this, it is interpretable as an exhortation to good mothering. The word 'parent' is gender-blind and obliterates oppressive imbalances in the roles and experience of mothers by

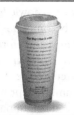

'The way I see it' slogan reads:

Every 20 minutes... less time than it will take you to drink your coffee, another child is diagnosed with autism. Learn the early warning signs of autism, and if you're concerned about your child's development, talk to your doctor. Early intervention could make a big difference to your child's future.

Figure 2.1 The Coffee Cup example: Starbucks Autism Awareness campaign.

using the gender-neutral language of 'parenting'.[41] In autism discourse, 'parent' is often a synonym for 'mother', because the vast majority of primary carers of autistic children are mothers. Studies of parental attitudes, parent-rated behaviour scales and parent-mediated interventions often overwhelmingly rely on mothers to participate. Good mothering tacitly means offering as much therapy as possible to the child, at the expense of any other career; Gil Eyal and colleagues[42] refers to this as the 'vocation' of autism parenting.

The threat of autism, this framing of risk, prompts anxiety which demands action. EIB targets the family, in partnership with medical institutions, as the site of early detection and intervention. Intervention may involve one-to-one teaching or up to 40 hours of speech, occupational and Applied Behavioural Analysis (ABA) therapies a week.[42] One US survey suggested parents use as many as 111 different therapies;[43] the mean number used at any one time was seven. The more severe the autism, the more types of treatments parents experimented with. In her work on attention deficit hyperactivity disorder (ADHD), Singh situates mothers' actions in the context of the multiple pressures they feel from so many sources, such as the Coffee Cup campaign.[44] A patriarchal culture that allows mothers to be culpable of their children's behaviour, responsible for monitoring the progress of the child and for 'doing something' if autism is detected, is a driver for the adoption of highly suspect therapies. The neurodiversity movement (Chapter 4) encourages better choices by situating autism as non-problematic – a condition that cannot, and perhaps should not, be 'fixed'.

The moral obligation for mothers to treat, monitor and report to clinicians is not new;[45] through a sociological lens, it is a form of surveillance medicine.[46,47] Surveillance medicine, the screening, monitoring and establishment of early risk factors, involves monitoring across a whole population, including healthy people.[46] Sociologists such as Ulrich Beck have pointed to a 'politics of anxiety' in the risk society.[48] David Armstrong writes about how infants were the first population to be scrutinised and surveyed for potential risks to normal childhood, such as being of a height and weight that fall outside statistical norms.[46]

Concepts of surveillance draw on Michel Foucault's work, particularly his book *Discipline and Punish*,[49] in which he describes how people are monitored, understood and regulated via institutions, which for babies include nurseries, research institutes, health visits and baby clinics. Foucault describes how people are first trained and observed in institutional settings to produce knowledge about disciplinary norms (for example, the observation of babies in maternity hospitals that produces knowledge about paediatrics, or the knowledge production of baby-sibs studies) and subsequently populations become monitored and subject to regulatory controls. Screening and surveillance therefore promote framing and recognition of differences as problems that were formerly not part of a medical remit. Hence, for good or ill, surveillance fosters medicalisation. The community is encouraged to monitor others in the community, providing normative standards of behaviour. This community policing and neighbourly surveillance were heightened during the 2020 Covid-19 lockdown to maintain social and behavioural norms.

Foucault wrote about the historical steps from a past model of external monitoring and top-down surveillance by powerful actors in the establishment, such as monarchs and lawyers, to community surveillance that provides a net-like power structure in which everyone is responsible for upholding normal behaviour, to the inculcation of internalised self-surveillance, the internalisation of bio-power, so that one comes to 'subjectivise' oneself and discipline one's own body.[49] Mothers' internalisation of vigilance and responsibility for the monitoring of their child seem to be an example of a relational form of bio-power.

In the case of the Coffee Cup, an exhortation for parents to perform surveillance of their child invokes anxiety, with autism described like a threatening disease. The Coffee Cup therefore promotes both pathologisation and vigilance and invokes autism as an object in itself, distant and removed from the individual person, meaning a person may become alienated from it.[50] For Foucault, a condition such as autism is objectified or 'spatialised' by its description as an entity that exists independently of the person (in texts and on coffee cups, etc.). Diagnosis locates autism in a second space, the brain, but autism also requires a third space, the social realm, because it is rendered in interaction. According to Foucault, 'truth' is produced through these levels of spatialisation, exercised by the professional gaze.[51] Once objectified, autism (or any condition) is subject to discipline, and through its control, subjection leads to the subjectification of people who are diagnosed. Although young children may not be able to resist this, adults can – a topic I will return to in Chapter 4. But Foucault was a master of the rhetorical device; others see power dynamics very differently, with less sinister overtones.

A similar rhetorical device to that of the Coffee Cup (risk, threat, requiring action) appears in most medical funding applications that try to identify early signs of autism. Research into either biomarkers or behavioural markers in infancy usually starts with a statement about autism's terrible impact on personal outcomes, families and the economy. Autism is often positioned as an object that is thoroughly bad news, the threat of which provokes anxiety and should be eliminated as early as possible.

Selective interpretation of data justifies the use of language to back up the EIB story, such as Green and colleagues' study of intervention for at-risk babies in which parents delivered the intervention.[52] Results were described as 'encouraging' despite there being no significant improvement in the primary outcome (attentiveness to parent); indeed, a few babies had a worse outcome. The abstract describes first how 'point estimates suggest the intervention increased the primary outcome of infant attentiveness', although qualifies this as 'including possibilities ranging from a small negative treatment effect to a strongly positive treatment effect' (actually it had a non-significant effect). The positioning and wording of reporting, in this and other literature, bolster the EIB narrative by accentuating the positive and diminishing the negative of EIB. Green and colleagues correctly reported the possibility of a negative outcome but the results were nevertheless framed as 'exciting' in the promise of intervention research.

Another example is a research paper, published in the journal *Autism*, that analysed the socio-demographic and child-based factors that predict late diagnosis.[26] The discussion describes how children are at risk of late diagnosis (after five years old): 'our understanding of "*red flags*" for *missed* diagnosis, that is early characteristics for children *at risk* of receiving a late diagnosis' (my italics). The phrase 'red flags' indicates autism is something that should raise an alarm and being 'at risk' of receiving a late diagnosis is troubling.

The Coffee Cup, and other forms of the EIB narrative, exhorts parents (specifically mothers) to perform surveillance and early childhood monitoring, to report proto-autism behaviours and, if possible, to intervene early. This surely leads to more early referrals and ultimately more diagnoses, contributing, perhaps in a small way, to autism's rise.

Caveats to EIB

There is a lack of evidence that diagnosis is stable at younger ages.[13] At very young ages, it is difficult to distinguish an autistic from an allistic (non-autistic) child, to distinguish a toddler who is not speaking because they may continue to display traits of autism later in life from a toddler who is a slow developer and will catch up. Some children grow out of autistic traits: 30% of children who are given a diagnosis at two years old no longer meet the criteria for an autism spectrum disorder (ASD) diagnosis at four.[53]

There is more uncertainty about future trajectories when screening procedures for autism begin before the child is two.[54] Our work followed the trajectories of two groups of children from two years old to 12; both groups were measured with comparably severe autistic-type traits at age two. The children in one group received an autism diagnosis, while those in the other did not.[55, 56] At adolescence, the children without an autism diagnosis were better on a range of outcomes. In other words, some pre-school-age children who have autistic traits can improve to sub-clinical levels without having ever been diagnosed or treated. In these cases, 'wait and see' may indeed be the best strategy.

To me, our work underlined that the human child is born in an immature state and learns adaptive behaviours as they grow. Many behaviours characteristic of developmental disorders are noticeable in all younger children: hand flapping, hyperactivity, inattention and motor difficulties are all common in toddlerhood. Resolving, at a very early stage, who has a lifelong impairment (and what impairment) and who will catch up is extremely difficult. In medical parlance, the specificity of these early signs in predicting autism may be very low, with many false positives. In a prospective Danish cohort of more than 75,000 children, in infancy the signs that distinguished autism from intellectual disability were unclear and at 18 months old, the positive predictive values (the probability that subjects with a positive test truly have autism) were below 10% for both individual predictors and aggregated risk scores.[57]

In addition, as children grow up the extent of autistic behaviours tends to diminish.[58] The age effect is illustrated by the seasonal influence on ADHD diagnosis. Summer-born children are more likely to be diagnosed with ADHD; a systematic review showed ADHD is consistently diagnosed more often in children who are young for their school year (which starts in the autumn in the UK),[59] not because they have more ADHD but simply because, relative to their peers, younger children display more behavioural characteristics of ADHD. Taking a developmental perspective therefore throws up challenges to the current recommendation for the reduction of age of diagnosis of autism to very young children.

Another counter to EIB is that diagnosis is not a neutral process of identification but shapes how others react to the baby. Given a specific childhood diagnosis, the people around the child (parents, teachers and clinicians), tend to interpret the child's behaviour in the diagnostic frame.[60] This may lead to an expectancy bias, in the classroom for example, that negatively affects outcomes.[61–63] Thus, very early labelling is problematic even if you consider a young baby either categorically has autism or does not, which is debatable. If the diagnosis is a false positive, those around the child might look at them through an autism lens; could this not negatively affect their trajectory?

Advocates of early diagnosis, on the other hand, see early identification as a crucial step to enable access to support and accommodations that benefit all children; diagnosis opens the gateways to intervention.[64] Autism can certainly act as an explanatory frame for differences in a child's biological and psychological make-up, which can radically improve the functioning of the family. As we have seen, autism researchers have emphasised the critical importance of intervening early in autistic children's lives to give them the best chance of meaningful communication.

A final caveat is that, despite the overwhelming call for early intervention, systematic reviews suggest research into early interventions is of poor quality and the effectiveness of early intervention is not proven for children with autism.[12] The rhetoric around early identification is widespread, and therefore should be underpinned by a rigorous evidence base. In fact, randomised controlled trials (RCTs) on early interventions are rare. One systematic review uncovered a replicated finding that many children who receive early intensive intervention, across methodologies, do *not* demonstrate dramatic gains in social, cognitive, adaptive and educational functioning or autism-specific behaviours.[12] A more recent review on the effects of ABA concluded there is weak or very weak evidence that ABA is a useful behavioural treatment for some children with autism and none that it alters core autism symptoms.[65]

The best that can be concluded is that some interventions improve some areas of functioning and sometimes improve cognition, in some young autistic children, some of the time. What is not often acknowledged is that early interventions for autism have high costs both for the children and in terms of parents' financial and time commitment. Programmes involving more than 40 hours of intensive therapy a week may be exhausting for parents (disproportionately mothers) and children alike.[42] The extra parenting work (usually mothering work) is implicitly expected to be done at home, even though a better outcome is not guaranteed. Nor is it currently possible for a clinician to confidently recommend a particular treatment for a particular child. There seems to be a disjunction between the level of actual evidence for the efficacy of early interventions for autism and what

I would term the rhetoric of early intervention and surveillance that designates good mothering.

Biomarkers

'At-risk' status can also be assigned from the evidence of biomarkers: objective, biological, measurable differences. For some conditions, biomarkers are physical attributes such as weight or heart rate; for autism, the biomarkers are usually neurological or genetic differences.

Some researchers use indices of risk or algorithms that calculate from a combination of biomarkers. For example, for ADHD, a genetic risk profile combines a number of genetic markers into an overall at-risk-of-ADHD score, a polygenic risk score.[66] In this way, researchers increase the predictive power of their models and, based on a risk index, can calculate a person's estimated probability of developing a condition. Considering an at-risk group in this way often gives access to larger and younger populations than would be possible if only confirmed cases were considered.

Perhaps the ultimate in baby surveillance is an electronic romper suit that monitors all aspects of the wearer's behaviour for 'warning' signs. In 2015, I interviewed a technology expert with many years' experience of designing computer algorithms to detect mouse movements in the laboratory. He described his company's on-going project to design romper suits to be used in the home to recognise the autism behavioural phenotype and help detect autism.[67] This 'smart' baby suit has sensors woven into the fabric that monitor the baby's heart rate, respiration, mobility and movement against normal parameters and automatically and securely transmit the data to the researchers' lab. The design was commissioned by at-risk-of-autism researchers but perhaps will be rolled out to the general population. Late development and missed milestones will ring 'alarm bells', raise 'red flags' and provide the required 'early warnings'.

For many years, there has been a push to detect biomarkers of autism because, as some argue, a biomarker is considered to be a more objective measure, and potentially a better mechanism of identification, than behavioural clinical assessments[68] which are subjective and dependent on the settings in which they are recorded. Plausible biomarkers for autism are measures such as brain circumference, genetic profile or a particular pattern of activity in the brain during a certain task, normally revealed by magnetic resonance imaging (MRI), but studies have identified many others.[69] Some scientists have advocated the fusing of behavioural definitions with biological, particularly neurological, indicators, for all psychiatric classes.[70] Perhaps, neither is 'better'; just different. Publicising, operationalising or adjusting either definitions or indicators will both influence our understanding of the autism category and alter who is in it. Autism is partly a product of how it is measured and identified.

In medical discourse, ethical arguments regarding 'at-risk' status are often founded on the notion of false positives. Statements about diagnosis and at-risk status use terms such as inaccuracy, misdiagnosis, false positive and validity. In this language, being named at-risk-of-autism may not *accurately* reflect your status (you may be a *false positive*), leading to *misdiagnosis* and raising questions about the *validity* of the at-risk category. These terms confer notions of 'truth', 'fact' and an 'objectivity' to be striven for. Again, these words assume there is a true fixed autism to be measured against and that conferring at-risk status does not in itself shape how we understand and define autism, how often we refer for autism and how deeming babies at risk could alter their developmental trajectory.

To take an example, let's say a neuro-marker is discovered, for example differences in white-matter tracts,[69] that forms a biomarker to identify autism. The at-risk group of babies thus identified will be a slightly different bunch to the babies identified as at risk by their behaviours, such as head lag. In this hypothetical example, publicising the neuro-work leads to understandings of autism as a neural condition (the white-matter tract difference). Atypical white-matter tract at-risk babies are more likely to be referred and diagnosed. Thus, the net effect of finding biomarkers contributes to what being 'at risk' of autism looks like, and who qualifies as having autism may be very slightly reshaped.

Although biomarker results are frequently described as 'promising', they are not often replicated or applicable to the whole spectrum. However, the search for genetic markers for autism has revealed some very useful markers of rare syndromes, for example Williams syndrome. The genetics of autism are complex, with different genetic sub-profiles that involve multi-faceted interactions with the environment.[71-73] Because what is diagnosable as autism is a slowly moving target, the search for a fixed set of biomarkers against which to compare is like having moving goalposts; it may be better to search for sub-groups across the spectrum. The latest iteration of the *Diagnostic and Statistical Manual of Mental Disorders* (DSM-5) has dropped the distinction between Asperger's disorder and autistic disorder but acknowledges differences within the autism spectrum, which is now stratified by the severity both of social communication impairment and restricted and repetitive patterns of behaviour, and with and without co-occurring intellectual disability. In DSM-5 the autism spectrum is also codified by known genetic conditions, biomarkers, although only a small percentage of cases have known genetic markers.

Despite the move towards sub-grouping, there is still investment in discovering the genetics of autism across the whole spectrum. Some research groups aspire to create a genetic test for autism that could be administered before birth, and some commercial laboratories offer parents a non-invasive pre-natal test they claim can screen for mutations in a range of genes, including some related to autism.[74] This claim has provoked an outraged reaction from the autistic community. In 2005, the autistic activist Meg Evans created the *Autistic Genocide Clock* as part of her *Star Trek* fanfiction website, *Ventura33*. Evans became mobilised after joining the autistic forum, *Aspergia*, and later the chatroom *Aspies for Freedom*, founded by Amy and Gareth Nelson, who also published a declaration that autistic people should be recognised as a minority group.[75] The *Autism Genocide Clock* was a ten-year countdown in the image of a clock; it responded to and resisted a pronouncement in 2005 that genetic research on autism could lead to a genetic test within ten years. Evans's point was that a pre-natal genetic test for autism could lead to abortions of foetuses that test positive for autism – in her view, a form of genocide. Writing in a collection of stories about autistic activists released as part of our *Exploring Diagnosis* project,[76] she described her timer clock as a reaction to autism discourse that, as she puts it, says 'the world should not have autistic people in it'. Evans took the clock down in 2011.

Certainly, the work towards pre-natal testing positions autism as a suitable rationale for abortion. Presumably such a test would be accompanied by genetic counselling for parents who chose to take it, to support them to decide whether to abort a baby with autism. Having been through such a scenario myself (when I was pregnant, my daughter screened positive for being at risk of Edwards's syndrome; it turned out to be a false positive), I know both how stressful this process can be for parents, and how powerful and potentially life changing the medical concepts can be in practice.

Evans's argument parallels those made by members of the disability rights movement, that pre-natal genetic tests are a form of eugenics, leading towards the elimination of people like them, and that allowing abortion on the grounds of disability is discriminatory.[77] Others argue quality of life is important to consider. Edward's syndrome leaves babies with heart, respiratory, kidney and gastrointestinal conditions, with 87% dying before one year old. The *Autistic Genocide Clock* illustrated the tension between a newer progressive, affirmative model of autism-as-identity and an older model of severe autism with co-morbidity and complications in a medical frame. Evans's strong language has parallels with historic resistance to the elimination of other minority groups.[78]

The twin processes of pushing back age of diagnosis into infancy and defining infants as 'at-risk' may have both contributed to the rise in autism observed in Chapter 1, if in a minor way. Earlier diagnosis contributes directly as a younger cohort is eligible for diagnosis. 'At -risk' status may contribute indirectly through widening 'what counts' as autism. Yet a more seismic shift in diagnostic practice occurred at the life stage covered in the next chapter: childhood.

References

1. Woods, J. J. & Wetherby, A. M. Early Identification of and Intervention for Infants and Toddlers Who Are at Risk for Autism Spectrum Disorder. *Lang. Speech Hear. Serv. Sch.* **34**, 180–193 (2003).
2. King, M. D., Fountain, C., Dakhlallah, D. & Bearman, P. S. Estimated Autism Risk and Older Reproductive Age. *Am. J. Public Health* **99**, 1673–1679 (2009).
3. Parner, E. T., Schendel, D. E. & Thorsen, P. Autism Prevalence Trends Over Time in Denmark: Changes in Prevalence and Age at Diagnosis. *Arch. Pediatr. Adolesc. Med.* **162**, 1150–1156 (2008).
4. Russell, G. *et al.* Time Trends in Autism Diagnosis Over 20 Years: A UK Population-based Cohort Study.
5. Ibañez, L. V., Grantz, C. J. & Messinger, D. S. The Development of Referential Communication and Autism Symptomatology in High-Risk Infants. *Infancy Off. J. Int. Soc. Infant Stud.* **18** (2013).

6. Teitelbaum, P., Teitelbaum, O., Nye, J., Fryman, J. & Maurer, R. G. Movement Analysis in Infancy may be Useful for Early Diagnosis of Autism. *Proc. Natl Acad. Sci. U. S. A.* **95**, 13982–13987 (1998).

7. Shen, M. D. & Piven, J. Brain and Behavior Development in Autism from Birth Through Infancy. *Dialogues Clin. Neurosci.* **19**, 325–333 (2017).

8. Jones, W. & Klin, A. Attention to Eyes is Present but in Decline in 2–6-Month-Old Infants Later Diagnosed with Autism. *Nature* **504**, 427–431 (2013).

9. Briggs, H. Autism Detectable 'in First Months'. *BBC News* 11 August (2013).

10. van Dijk, W., Faber, M. J., Tanke, M. A. C., Jeurissen, P. P. T. & Westert, G. P. Medicalisation and Overdiagnosis: What Society Does to Medicine. *Int. J. Health Policy Manag.* **5**, 619–622 (2016).

11. Clark, M. L. E., Vinen, Z., Barbaro, J. & Dissanayake, C. School Age Outcomes of Children Diagnosed Early and Later with Autism Spectrum Disorder. *J. Autism Dev. Disord.* **48**, 92–102 (2018).

12. Warren, Z. *et al.* A Systematic Review of Early Intensive Intervention for Autism Spectrum Disorders. *Pediatrics* **127**, e1303–e1311 (2011).

13. Allaby, D. M. & Sharma, D. M. Screening for Autism Spectrum Disorders in Children Below the Age of 5 years. A Draft Report for the UK National Screening Committee. Solutions for Public Health. (2011).

14. Chen, I. Understanding Autism: Baby Steps. *Spectrum | Autism Research News.* www.spectrumnews.org/features/deep-dive/what-baby-siblings-can-teach-us-about-autism/ (2017).

15. Bumiller, K. The Geneticization of Autism: From New Reproductive Technologies to the Conception of Genetic Normalcy. *Signs J. Women Cult. Soc.* **34**, 875–899 (2009).

16. Giovanni, M. A. *et al.* Health-care Referrals from Direct-to-consumer Genetic Testing. *Genet. Test. Mol. Biomark.* **14**, 817–819 (2010).

17. Hedgecoe, A. Schizophrenia and the Narrative of Enlightened Geneticization. *Soc. Stud. Sci.* **31**, 875–911 (2001).

18. Latimer, J. *The Gene, the Clinic, and the Family: Diagnosing Dysmorphology, Reviving Medical Dominance* (Routledge, 2013).

19. Folstein, S. & Rutter, M. Infantile Autism: A Genetic Study of 21 Twin Pairs. *J. Child Psychol. Psychiatry* **18**, 297–321 (1977).

20. Sandin, S. *et al.* The Familial Risk of Autism. *JAMA* **311**, 1770–1777 (2014).

21. Brett, D., Warnell, F., McConachie, H. & Parr, J. R. Factors Affecting Age at ASD Diagnosis in UK: No Evidence that Diagnosis Age has Decreased Between 2004 and 2014. *J. Autism Dev. Disord.* **46**, 1974–1984 (2016).

22. Daniels, A. M. & Mandell, D. S. Explaining Differences in Age at Autism Spectrum Disorder Diagnosis: A Critical Review. *Autism Int. J. Res. Pract.* **18**, 583–597 (2014).

23. Shattuck, P. T. *et al.* Timing of Identification Among Children with an Autism Spectrum Disorder: Findings from a Population-based Surveillance Study. *J. Am. Acad. Child Adolesc. Psychiatry* **48**, 474–483 (2009).

24. Sheldrick, R. C., Maye, M. P. & Carter, A. S. Age at First Identification of Autism Spectrum Disorder: An Analysis of Two US Surveys. *J. Am. Acad. Child Adolesc. Psychiatry* **56**, 313–320 (2017).

25. Zwaigenbaum, L. *et al.* Developmental Functioning and Symptom Severity Influence Age of Diagnosis in Canadian Preschool Children with Autism. *Paediatr. Child Health* **24**, e57–e65 (2019).

26. Hosozawa, M. *et al.* Determinants of an Autism Spectrum Disorder Diagnosis in Childhood and Adolescence: Evidence from the UK Millennium Cohort Study. *Autism Int. J. Res. Pract.* 24, 1557–1565 (2020) doi:10.1177/1362361320913671.

27. Sivberg, B. Parents' Detection of Early Signs in their Children Having an Autistic Spectrum Disorder. *J. Pediatr. Nurs.* 18, 433–439 (2003).

28. Gliga, T., Jones, E. J. H., Bedford, R., Charman, T. & Johnson, M. H. From Early Markers to Neuro-developmental Mechanisms of Autism. *Dev. Rev.* 34, 189–207 (2014).

29. Landa, R. J. Diagnosis of Autism Spectrum Disorders in the first 3 Years of Life. *Nat. Clin. Pract. Neurol.* 4, 138–147 (2008).

30. Baranek, G. T. Autism During Infancy: A Retrospective Video Analysis of Sensory-motor and Social Behaviors at 9–12 Months of Age. *J. Autism Dev. Disord.* 29, 213–224 (1999).

31. Le Couteur, A. *et al.* A Broader Phenotype of Autism: The Clinical Spectrum in Twins. *J. Child Psychol. Psychiatry* 37, 785–801 (1996).

32. Mulligan, S. & White, B. P. Sensory and Motor Behaviors of Infant Siblings of Children with and Without Autism. *Am. J. Occup. Ther. Off. Publ. Am. Occup. Ther. Assoc.* 66, 556–566 (2012).

33. Gallagher, S. & Varga, S. Conceptual Issues in Autism Spectrum Disorders. *Curr. Opin. Psychiatry* 28, 127–132 (2015).

34. LeBarton, E. S. & Iverson, J. M. Fine Motor Skill Predicts Expressive Language in Infant Siblings of Children with Autism. *Dev. Sci.* 16, 815–827 (2013).

35. Sacrey, L.-A. R., Bennett, J. A. & Zwaigenbaum, L. Early Infant Development and Intervention for Autism Spectrum Disorder. *J. Child Neurol.* 30, 1921–1929 (2015).

36. Leonard, H. C., Elsabbagh, M., Hill, E. L. & Basis Team. Early and Persistent Motor Delay in Infants at-risk of Developing Autism Spectrum Disorder: A Prospective Study. *Eur. J. Dev. Psychol.* 11, 18–35 (2014).

37. Nickel, L. R., Thatcher, A. R., Keller, F., Wozniak, R. H. & Iverson, J. M. Posture Development in Infants at Heightened vs. Low Risk for Autism Spectrum Disorders. *Infancy Off. J. Int. Soc. Infant Stud.* 18, 639–661 (2013).

38. Watson, L. R. *et al.* The First Year Inventory: Retrospective Parent Responses to a Questionnaire Designed to Identify One-year-olds at Risk for Autism. *J. Autism Dev. Disord.* 37, 49–61 (2007).

39. Wallace, S., Parr, J. & Herd, A. One in a Hundred. www.autistica.org.uk/wp-content/uploads/2014/10/One-in-a-Hundred-Autisticas-Report.pdf (2012).

40. McGuire, A. E. Buying Time: The S/pace of Advocacy and the Cultural Production of Autism. *Can. J. Disabil. Stud.* 2, 98–125 (2013).

41. Traustadottir, R. Mothers Who Care. *J. Fam. Issues* 12, 211–228 (1991).

42. Eyal, G., Hart, B., Onculer, E., Neta, O. & Rossi, N. *The Autism Matrix* (Polity, 2010).

43. Green, V. A. *et al.* Internet Survey of Treatments Used by Parents of Children with Autism. *Res. Dev. Disabil.* 27, 70–84 (2006).

44. Singh, I. Doing Their Jobs: Mothering with Ritalin in a Culture of Mother-blame. *Soc. Sci. Med.* 59, 1193–1205 (2004).

45. Nadesan, M. *Constructing Autism: Unravelling the 'Truth' and Understanding the Social* (Routledge, 2005).

46. Armstrong, D. The Rise of Surveillance Medicine. *Sociol. Health Illn.* 17, 393–404 (1995).

47. Armstrong, L. *And They Call It Help: The Psychiatric Policing of America's Children* (Addison-Wesley, 1993).

48. Beck, U. *Risk Society: Towards a New Modernity* (Sage, 1992).

49. Foucault, M. *Discipline and Punish: The Birth of the Prison* (Vintage, 1995).

50. Taussig, M. T. Reification and the Consciousness of the Patient. *Soc. Sci. Med. [B]* 14, 3–13 (1980).

51. Vakirtzi, E. & Bayliss, P. Towards a Foucauldian Methodology in the Study of Autism: Issues of Archaeology, Genealogy, and Subjectification. *J. Philos. Educ.* 47, 364–378 (2013).

52. Green, J. *et al.* Parent-mediated Intervention Versus no Intervention for Infants at High Risk of Autism: A Parallel, Single-blind, Randomised Trial. *Lancet Psychiatry* 2, 133–140 (2015).

53. Turner, L. M. & Stone, W. L. Variability in Outcome for Children with an ASD Diagnosis at Age 2. *J. Child Psychol. Psychiatry* 48, 793–802 (2007).

54. Rutter, M. Autism: Its Recognition, Early Diagnosis, and Service Implications. *J. Dev. Behav. Pediatr. JDBP* 27, S54–S58 (2006).

55. Russell, G., Ford, T., Steer, C. & Golding, J. Identification of Children with the Same Level of Impairment as Children on the Autistic Spectrum, and Analysis of their Service Use. *J. Child Psychol. Psychiatry* 51, 643–651 (2010).

56. Russell, G. *et al.* Social and Behavioural Outcomes in Children Diagnosed with Autism Spectrum Disorders: A Longitudinal Cohort Study. *J. Child Psychol. Psychiatry* 53, 735–744 (2012).

57. Lemcke, S., Juul, S., Parner, E. T., Lauritsen, M. B. & Thorsen, P. Early Signs of Autism in Toddlers: A Follow-up Study in the Danish National Birth Cohort. *J. Autism Dev. Disord.* 43, 2366–2375 (2013).

58. Shattuck, P. T. *et al.* Change in Autism Symptoms and Maladaptive Behaviors in Adolescents and Adults with an Autism Spectrum Disorder. *J. Autism Dev. Disord.* 37, 1735–1747 (2007).

59. Whitely, M. *et al.* Attention Deficit Hyperactivity Disorder Late Birthdate Effect Common in Both High and Low Prescribing International Jurisdictions: A Systematic Review. *J. Child Psychol. Psychiatry* 60, 380–391 (2019).

60. Fogel, L. S. & Nelson, R. O. The Effects of Special Education Labels on Teachers. *J. Sch. Psychol.* 21, 241–251 (1983).

61. Jussim, L. Self-Fulfilling Prophecies: A Theoretical and Integrative Review. *Psychol. Rev.* 93, 429–445 (1986).

62. Jussim, L., Palumbo, P., Chatman, C., Madon, S. & Smith, A. Stigma and Self-fulfilling Prophecies. *Soc. Psychol. Stigma* 374–418 (2000).

63. Rosenthal, R. & Jacobson, L. Teachers' Expectancies: Determinants of Pupils' IQ Gains. *Psychol. Rep.* 19, 115–118 (1966).

64. Crais, E. R., Watson, L. R., Baranek, G. T. & Reznick, J. S. Early Identification of Autism: How Early Can We Go? *Semin. Speech Lang.* 27, 143–160 (2006).

65. Reichow, B., Hume, K., Barton, E. E. & Boyd, B. A. Early Intensive Behavioral Intervention (EIBI) for Young Children with Autism Spectrum Disorders (ASD). *Cochrane Database Syst. Rev.* doi:10.1002/14651858.CD009260.pub3 (2018).

66. Brikell, I. *et al.* The Contribution of Common Genetic Risk Variants for ADHD to a General Factor of Childhood Psychopathology. *Mol. Psychiatry* 1–13 (2018) doi:10.1038/s41380-018-0109-2.

67. Noldus. Aims-2-trials. www.noldus.com/projects/aims-2-trials (2015).

68. Atkinson, A. *et al.* NIH Biomarkers Definitions Working Group Biomarkers and Surrogate Endpoints: Preferred Definitions and Conceptual Framework. *Clin. Pharmacol. Ther.* **69**, 89–95 (2001).

69. Wolff, J. J. *et al.* Differences in White Matter Fiber Tract Development Present from 6 to 24 Months in Infants with Autism. *Am. J. Psychiatry* **169**, 589–600 (2012).

70. Zeman, A. Neurology is Psychiatry – and Vice Versa. *Pract. Neurol.* **14**, 136–144 (2014).

71. Folstein, S. E. & Rosen-Sheidley, B. Genetics of Autism: Complex Aetiology for a Heterogeneous Disorder. *Nat. Rev. Genet.* **2**, 943–955 (2001).

72. Persico, A. M. & Napolioni, V. Autism Genetics. *Behav. Brain Res.* **251**, 95–112 (2013).

73. Yang, M. S. & Gill, M. A Review of Gene Linkage, Association and Expression Studies in Autism and an Assessment of Convergent Evidence. *Int. J. Dev. Neurosci. Off. J. Int. Soc. Dev. Neurosci.* **25**, 69–85 (2007).

74. The Problems with Prenatal Testing for Autism. *Spectrum | Autism Research News.* www.spectrumnews.org/features/deep-dive/the-problems-with-prenatal-testing-for-autism/ (2019).

75. Nelson, A. Declaration From the Autism Community That They Are a Minority Group. www.prweb.com/releases/2004/11/prweb179444.htm (2004).

76. Kapp, S. K. *Autistic Community and the Neurodiversity Movement: Stories from the Frontline* (Springer Singapore, 2020).

77. Woman with Down's Syndrome Takes UK Govt to Court Over Allowing Abortion up to Birth for Disabilities. *Right To Life UK* https://righttolife.org.uk/news/woman-with-downs-syndrome-takes-uk-govt-to-court-over-allowing-abortion-up-to-birth-for-disabilities/ (2020).

78. Dyck, E. & Russell, G. Challenging Psychiatric Classification: Healthy Autistic Diversity the Neurodiversity Movement. In *Mental Health in Historical Perspective: Healthy Minds in the Twentieth Century* (eds. Taylor, S. J. & Brumby, A.) (Palgrave MacMillan, 2020).

3 Children

Childhood

Since it was first introduced as a diagnostic class, autism has been thought of as a disorder of childhood. In higher-income countries, most autism diagnoses are made when children are between three and ten years old, the early to mid-childhood period.[1-3] Developmental psychologists tend to approach childhood as one of a series of pre-determined stages (infancy, childhood, adolescence), in which developmental milestones such as language acquisition, awareness of self and the ability to attribute mental states to others occur, milestones that are recorded as absent or delayed in children with autism. This view of developmental milestones at fixed stages of development harks back to the Swiss psychologist, Jean Piaget's, work in the 1930s, a universalist view that early human life stages follow the same pattern everywhere and, if not, there is aberrant development.[4]

Defining what achievements are characteristic of a given developmental stage or age band operates in a somewhat context-free model. Talcot Parsons, and other sociologists of the post-war period, brought the child's environment to the fore, introducing the idea of socialisation.[5] Socialisation takes place in a child's expanding sphere of influence; for tiny babies, the mother; as the maturing infant's horizons expand, the family; for children in schools and for adolescents, peer groups. Resistance, like youth subculture, was often viewed as socialisation gone wrong. An autistic trait, in this light, is the inability to be socialised or to grasp rules inculcated through socialisation.

Madeleine Leonard gives a historical account of the sociology of childhood.[4] She describes how, in the 1980s, the top-down idea of children as passive sponges soaking up social messages was challenged by sociologists. They countered that childhood is itself a construct, in which the child influences all aspects of their environment as well as being influenced by it;[5] the everyday lives of children should be the focus of research, not just the 'deviance' of developmental psycho-pathology.[6] She describes how schools were painted by neo-Marxists as places to learn the value of oneself in terms of being a future productive worker and to be taught that 'people who work with brains are paid more and valued more than people who work with hands'. That is, schools are sites of children's socialisation, places that instil and establish inequalities.

The concept of autism as a category has radically shifted in the same time span as these revisions to our ideas about childhood. Originally described in 1943, autism was thought of as a form of child schizophrenia throughout the 1960s and 1970s. The third edition of the *Diagnostic and Statistical Manual of Mental Disorders* (DSM-III), published in 1980, established autism as a separate diagnosis and described it as a 'pervasive developmental disorder', distinct from schizophrenia. DSM-III was revised in 1987, significantly altering the autism criteria. It broadened the concept of autism by adding a diagnosis (pervasive developmental disorder not otherwise specified, PDD-NOS) at the mild end of the spectrum and dropping the requirement for onset before 30 months. Both DSM and the *International Classification of Disease* (ICD) expanded their definitions of autism spectrum disorder in the 1990s to include Asperger's syndrome or Asperger's disorder, meaning that children with typical and above-average intellectual ability were included. DSM-IV, released in 1994 and revised in 2000, was the first edition to categorise autism as a spectrum.

As a consequence, over the last 20 years in high-income countries, there has been an increased and ongoing application of autism diagnoses to children of normal and above-average intelligence. In the USA, the modern shift from a predominantly 'lower-functioning' autistic child population to a 'higher-functioning' one has been documented in a sequential cohort study, published in 2012, of more than six million children in California.[7] This work reported an overall upward time trend, from 1994 to 2003, for any autism diagnosis. It was striking that the odds of autism diagnosis were 15 times greater for 'high-functioning' children in 2002 compared to 1992, whereas the odds of diagnosis increased only four-fold for the 'lower-functioning' group. Clearly, diagnosis of the group of children at the higher-functioning end of the spectrum is a driver of the dramatic rising trend in identification and diagnosis of autism.

A study in Sweden found that children aged seven to 12 years old who received a diagnosis of autism in 2014 had a 50% lower autism symptom score than did those diagnosed in 2004, whereas the diagnosis of autism simultaneously increased five-fold. They concluded that less severe autism symptoms have been required for diagnosis as time has passed.[8]

Figure 3.1 shows autistic traits in the whole population, including the sub-clinical population called the broad autism phenotype (BAP);[9] as already shown, autistic traits are roughly normally distributed.[10] The arrows illustrate the threshold for diagnosis moving to the left over time, and with time, more children included in the diagnosable tail of the distribution. The key point is that even a minor shift of threshold for diagnosis to the left, moving less severe cases into the mainstream 'threshold' region, means a much bigger jump in the proportion of children who become 'diagnosable'. This is because the new bars that are encompassed each contain a larger percentage of the population, hence the exponential rise in diagnosis. Note, that although the distribution bars are derived from our study,[11] the diagnostic threshold lines are there to illustrate the point and are not based on any real data.

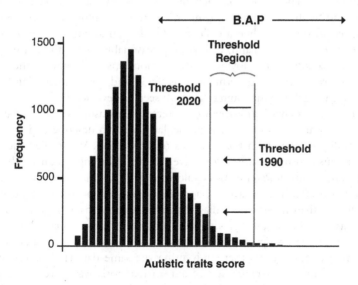

Figure 3.1 Changing boundary for diagnosis in children.

A paper in *JAMA Psychiatry*, published in 2019, provided a meta-analysis of studies between 1966 and 2019 and suggests that differences between people with autism diagnosis and those without have decreased over time, on average. The constructs the study measured, such as emotion recognition, theory of mind and brain size, had become nearer to the typical in the diagnosed group, or nearer the mean values in a population-based histogram. The authors suggested that changes in the definition of autism, from a narrowly defined and homogeneous population toward an inclusive and heterogeneous population, may reduce our capacity to build mechanistic models of the condition.[12]

Functioning

In medicine, functional impairment refers to limits due to an illness; functions in their daily lives that people with a disease cannot carry out. For young children with autism, functioning means the ability to carry out everyday tasks, such as getting dressed, cleaning their teeth, mixing with peers at school, eating, learning, communicating and taking an active part in family life. For adolescents, functioning might be indicated by mixing with peers, buying things in shops, tidying, maintaining personal hygiene and general life skills. Clearly, measuring functioning is mixed with social norms, particularly the idea of reaching milestones at certain ages/developmental stages. As level of functioning is adaptive it can't really be considered an individual characteristic, because one's ability to function is completely dependent on what one is required to do, one's support and one's circumstances.[13] There has been debate about the overlap between Asperger's disorder and 'high-functioning autism'; the latter is an informal diagnosis sometimes given in the UK when a child or adult has an average or above-average intelligence quotient (IQ) and/or is coping reasonably well with life issues such as housing, school or employment and relationships.[14,15] Some in the autistic community resist the use of terms such as 'high' and 'low'-functioning because people given the 'low-functioning' label are seen as devalued.[16]

Nevertheless, a child's *functioning* is a term and measure widely used in child psychiatry. In autism research it is particularly used to describe and quantify a child's ability to cope with the demands of daily living. We studied the age at which various autism diagnoses were given in the UK using data from the Avon Longitudinal Study of Parents And Children (ALSPAC).[3] Perhaps unsurprisingly, we found a markedly older average age of diagnosis for people with a diagnosis of Asperger's than those with a diagnosis of infantile autism (Figure 3.2). This implies (as do other studies) that age of diagnosis of autism in childhood is typically later for the group of children with autism who do not have an intellectual disability (ID). In another study using the same dataset, Colin Steer and colleagues found the average age of autism diagnosis was lower for children with more severe autistic traits.[10] As noted in Chapter 2, children who have a lower IQ and very severe autistic behaviour or who do not meet early developmental milestones as expected are probably going to be referred earlier in their life. Their parents and carers are likely to reach out for medical and educational help sooner than parents whose children are nearer the threshold, whose intellect is above average and whose language, although it may be idiosyncratic, is

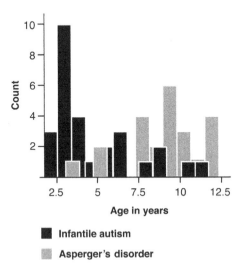

Figure 3.2 The average age of autism diagnosis in the Avon Longitudinal Study of Parents And Children (ALSPAC) dataset.

developed and allows the children to cope in early-years settings, which tend to be less demanding.

Although there is not a perfect mapping between functioning and IQ, the inter-relationship between IQ, autism severity, setting, support and demand, all play a role in determining good functioning.[17] Adaptive functioning (how well one copes or deals with various day-to-day tasks) has been strongly correlated with IQ in some autism studies, especially in the work of Susana Mouga and colleagues.[18] Their work, in which adaptive functioning has been associated with cognitive ability, suggests lower IQ means less success in learning to cope with the demands of everyday life although this does not speak to the quality of life more generally.[18]

Children present for diagnosis in later childhood when their behaviours become problematic as 'social demands exceed limited capacities', according to DSM-5.[19] This change may be due to changes in circumstances, such as moving to a new school.[20] Our analysis of attention deficit hyperactivity disorder (ADHD) diagnoses in the UK showed a distinct spike during the period of transition from primary to secondary school,[21] presumably because parents wanted more support for their children in the less-supported learning environment of secondary school. This is reminiscent of the Foucauldian 'surface of emergence'[22] – the field in which an object first arises. Foucault writes that pre-existing fields, such as family, social group or school, are always normative to some degree and will have developed a 'margin of tolerance' that roughly defines the field of what it considers unaccept-able.[22] The field may be secondary school, the object is diagnosable autism, because for an autism diagnosis to be considered there must be a negative impact on children and their carers; perhaps a child's behaviour only becomes problematic in the secondary school environment, where there are more demands. Between younger childhood, older childhood and adolescent childhood groups, it was in secondary school-aged children, that we saw the biggest increases in the recording of new autism diagnosis between 1998 and 2018 (see Figure 4.1).

In another study we conducted, parents reported their autistic children 'holding it together' and behaving well at school but, due to the intense effort needed,[23] 'melting down' when they returned home. In the threshold region (Figure 3.2), located at the boundary between sub-clinical and clinical, there are clearly circumstances that are more difficult (school is more demanding than home) and consequently children learn to 'mask' more. (Masking is the use of rote or learned behaviours and speech to cover up difficulties with social interaction, discussed further in Chapter 5.) There seems to be an interaction between biology, level of functioning, social expectation, masking and diagnosis. The issues of when and where diagnosis is rendered necessary raise questions about whether autism can be located in an individual person or only in interaction.

The lobbying and organisation of the various neuro-tribes are partly what have driven the shift of diagnostic threshold to the left in Figure 3.1, to older children.[24,25] Milder traits before secondary school may not have been considered diagnosable as an autism spectrum disorder before 1990, but later diagnosis is arguably a good way for a wider range of older children to access much-needed support and understanding. Some have argued that, if resources are scarce, the broader diagnosis may become an issue, because more diagnoses creates greater pressure on resources in health, education and other services, leading to a displacement of services from those who need them most.[26] A counter policy argument might be to target support for all people who struggle, and want a diagnosis, perhaps deflecting money from areas other than health. In other words, expanding the services 'pot' where there is more diagnosis, rather than leaving the size of the pot unchanged.

Looping

Looping is the idea that the diagnostic classifications we use to define illness (and other sorts of categories) can transform the people in the classified populations and they in turn can transform our understanding of the categories (Figure 3.3).[27] Ian Hacking, who writes somewhat rambling but brilliant philosophy papers in the *London Review of Books* among other places,[27,28] has written about autism several times. Hacking's original idea was that looping in diagnosis entails feedback operating through the patient's and others' self-awareness and shifts in their behaviour. The diagnostic category into which patients are grouped leads patients to reflect on themselves differently and others to treat them in a different way. Being classified as 'autistic' changes how a person acts and how others perceive them. People familiar with psychology and sociology, especially those familiar with Howard Becker on labelling theory[29] and Robert Merton's theory of self-fulfilling prophecies,[30] which sparked more than 50 years of empirical research,[31] might suggest Hacking is re-inventing the wheel, or rather the 'loop'. However, these theories concern people who are labelled (for example, by diagnosis) and how diagnostic labels can transform identities and outcomes. Hacking's looping covers these aspects but has an additional focus on how the *diagnostic category itself* and scientific classification may be transformed by the actions of those who are labelled (Figure 3.3).

Hacking writes about the concept of 'human kinds' in classifications such as 'autism'. Unlike 'natural kinds' (for example, 'stones'), these are classes that are themselves altered by the act of classification. Autism, or any other diagnostic class, is a 'human kind', demarcated by its shifting through its classification.[32] For Hacking, looping means that diagnostic categories are 'moving targets' and their

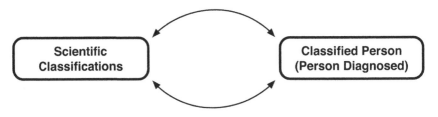

Figure 3.3 Hacking's early ideas about looping.

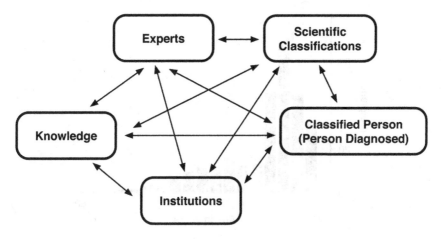

Figure 3.4 Hacking's later ideas about looping (adapted from Tekin).

reification as static objects is misplaced. There is plenty of highly technical debate in philosophy about the notions of 'kinds', of which I understand little. Luckily, this is not my concern here.

In later work, Hacking described a more complicated model.[28] As configured by Serife Tekin,[33] Hacking's revised model is less of a loop; rather, all points influence all others (Figure 3.4). In this model the category (such as autism) is in a constant flux of remaking through negotiations among scientific experts, people with autism, parents and professionals – an interplay of *social movements, health institutions* and *scientific experts* that creates and shapes our *knowledge*, diagnostic *classification* and 'how we view autistic people and ultimately how we understand autism'.[34] One problem with this model is that it puts knowledge in one homogenous box, begging the question of whose knowledge and whose understanding. Others have criticised Hacking's ideas because it is not clear how much patients' shifted behaviour and self-awareness might be due to the act of labelling, how much to the consequences of labelling (such as treatments) and how much to the progress of the condition.

The review we conducted, which covered all the autism research published in 12 months in high-impact autism-specific journals, provides a candidate looping effect. We wanted to find out whether most autistic participants who took part in autism research studies had either an IQ in the normal range or an intellectual disability. The review included more than 300 autism studies, which together had recruited more than 100,000 participants with autism. In 75% of the studies, the average age (Figure 3.5) of participants with autism was under 20 years old, meaning the majority of autism research was conducted on or with children and adolescents. Moreover, you will recall (see Introduction, Figure 1) that we found only a handful of published autism studies from South America or Africa; more than 95% were from European or anglophone countries.

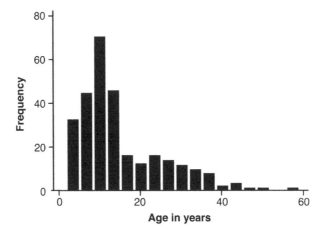

Figure 3.5 Mean age in years of participants with autism by frequency of study.

Bias and looping

We found that, across all autism studies, only about 6% of participants with autism had ID; in other words, approximately 94% of people participating in this sample of autism research did not. If researchers were aiming to create a representative sample of the population with autism according to published prevalence estimates,[35] each study should have had a stratified autism sample, with around 50% of participants with ID. These autism research studies therefore showed a selection bias against autistic participants with ID.[36] This phenomenon has been documented elsewhere: in the US National Database of Autism Research, which has 47,400 participants, only 11% have either ID or a borderline ID (an IQ below 85).

The causes of the ID bias are easy to identify. Research instruments are rarely designed for people with severe to profound ID, who may not readily understand research protocols and the potential benefits of participation, making it more difficult to obtain their informed consent to participate. And parents caring for an autistic child with ID have little time or energy to participate in research. Verbally fluent participants are easier to recruit for trials and other forms of research; we estimated the proportion of non- or minimally verbal autistic participants to be even smaller, just 2% of the pooled sample of participants.

Perhaps the most interesting aspect of our review was the way that the knowledge generated by the studies included was passed on. Ninety per cent of authors who cited the 300 studies included in our review applied the knowledge generated to the entire autism spectrum. Even studies that did not include *any* participants with ID were cited as if they applied to the entire autism spectrum. Daisy Elliott, a gifted member of our team, established this by meticulously tracking and checking citations of the studies we reviewed. Daisy's findings reflect how busy scientists operate, how science is done, how citations are frequently made after reading only the paper's abstract. Her work illustrated how 'facts' travel and how autism *knowledge* is primarily drawn from participants with specific profiles. It was clear there were inherent biases in the characteristics of who participated in published research studies about autism, who they were and where they came from. To return to looping effects, if the participants were primarily intellectually able, verbal children and adolescents (I shall call them IVCAs) from high-income, largely anglophone countries, then this profile underscores the research evidence base which in turn informs the diagnostic criteria.

Referring to the revised model of looping (Figure 3.4), one way in which diagnostic categories shift over time is through revisions to diagnostic criteria, such as the DSM and ICD. Revisions are discussed and implemented by work groups, using an evidence-based approach, assessing the strongest and latest research evidence to determine tweaks to the parameters of the category. Every family of medical diagnoses has its own specific work group, formed of the most respected *scientific experts* in their field, who undertake the highest-impact studies. For autism, the neurodevelopmental work group that revised the DSM-5 criteria published in 2013 comprised a band of eminent professors considered to be the authorities in autism research. This evidence-based process means, in theory, that the best scientific research-based evidence is used to construct and refine the diagnostic delineations of disease and disorder. Of course, the experts are also subject to lobbying from various mobilised tribes, as for any diagnosis.[37]

In this example, the American Psychiatric Association, which commissions the DSM, is the *institution* in Figure 3.4. As research evidence underpins any changes to the criteria, looping could occur if autistic people with ID are under-represented in the evidence base, assuming they have differing phenotypic and aetiological profiles from IVCAs. If IVCAs with autism are over-represented in research studies, the evidence base will reflect the characteristics of IVCAs and *knowledge* about autism will be mostly drawn from IVCA profile. Selection bias will lead to slight shifts in the definition of the category, as new knowledge and new criteria consequently emphasise the characteristics of IVCAs. Changes to the *classification* of autism, in turn, alter who is eligible for diagnosis. The new shape and boundaries of the category, who it contains, determine who will be eligible to participate in future autism research studies. And so the loop continues (Figure 3.6). Unlike Hacking's classic earlier description, this type of looping does not require a person to alter their behaviour because they are so classified.

This presumed loop (Figure 3.6) could lead to an entrenchment of autism as a condition most common in children with typical or above-average IQ. As there are many more children who have typical IQ than those who do not, the net effect of selection bias on ID loop could be to broaden the pool of children who are eligible for diagnosis.

The description of autism that encompasses people with above-average IQ has produced a range of cultural representations in high-income countries, ranging from children's television classics such as *Sesame Street* to the Scandi-noir thriller *The Bridge*. Fictional accounts, such as *The Curious Incident of the Dog in the*

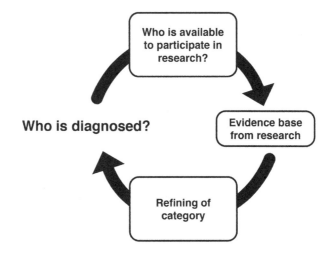

Figure 3.6 Schematic representation of looping effect.

Night-time, have been adapted into hit plays and, in cinema, autistic characters are common. First-wave autistic autobiographies, such as Donna Williams's *Nobody Nowhere*,[38] Temple Grandin's *Emergence*[39] and Oliver Sacks's account of their meeting in *An Anthropologist on Mars*,[40] have led to an explosion in so-called 'autie-biography'. Through autie-biography, adults without ID have become the most obvious voices of lived experience. Such works are discussed by Hacking as a route to access the experience of autism in a new way, leading to a new type of person.[41] And increasingly, these autism stories provide an accessible and powerful lens to explain differences in adults, as well as in children.

References

1. Hrdlicka, M. *et al.* Age at Diagnosis of Autism Spectrum Disorders: Is There an Association with Socioeconomic Status and Family Self-education About Autism? *Neuropsychiatr. Dis. Treat.* **12**, 1639–1644 (2016).
2. Mandell, D. S., Novak, M. M. & Zubritsky, C. D. Factors Associated With Age of Diagnosis Among Children With Autism Spectrum Disorders. *Pediatrics* **116**, 1480–1486 (2005).
3. Russell, G., Ford, T., Steer, C. & Golding, J. Identification of Children with the Same Level of Impairment as Children on the Autistic Spectrum, and Analysis of their Service Use. *J. Child Psychol. Psychiatry* **51**, 643–651 (2010).
4. Leonard, M. *The Sociology of Children, Childhood and Generation* (SAGE, 2015).
5. Bales, R. F. & Parsons, T. *Family: Socialization and Interaction Process* (Routledge, 1998).
6. Prout, A. & James, A. A New Paradigm for the Sociology of Childhood? Provenance, Promise and Problems. In *Constructing and Reconstructing Childhood* (ed. James, A. & Prout, A.) 6–28 (Taylor & Francis 2015).

7. Keyes, K. M. *et al.* Cohort Effects Explain the Increase in Autism Diagnosis Among Children Born from 1992 to 2003 in California. *Int. J. Epidemiol.* **41**, 495–503 (2012).

8. Arvidsson, O., Gillberg, C., Lichtenstein, P. & Lundström, S. Secular Changes in the Symptom Level of Clinically Diagnosed Autism. *J. Child Psychol. Psychiatry* **59**, 744–751 (2018).

9. Lainhart, J. E. *et al.* Autism, Regression, and the Broader Autism Phenotype. *Am. J. Med. Genet.* **113**, 231–237 (2002).

10. Steer, C. D., Golding, J. & Bolton, P. F. Traits Contributing to the Autistic Spectrum. *PLoS One* **5**, e12633 (2010).

11. Russell, G., Collishaw, S., Golding, J., Kelly, S. E. & Ford, T. Changes in Diagnosis Rates and Behavioural Traits of Autism Spectrum Disorders Over Time. *BJPsych Open* **1**(2), 110–115 (2015).

12. Rødgaard, E.-M., Jensen, K., Vergnes, J.-N., Soulières, I. & Mottron, L. Temporal Changes in Effect Sizes of Studies Comparing Individuals With and Without Autism: A Meta-analysis. *JAMA Psychiatry* **76**, 1124–1132 (2019).

13. World Health Organization. *International Classification of Functioning, Disability and Health* (WHO, 2004).

14. Gillberg, C. Asperger Syndrome and High-functioning Autism. *Br. J. Psychiatry* **172**, 200–209 (1998).

15. Ghaziuddin, M. & Mountain-Kimchi, K. Defining the Intellectual Profile of Asperger Syndrome: Comparison with High-functioning Autism. *J. Autism Dev. Disord.* **34**, 279–284 (2004).

16. Kapp, S. K. Social Support, Well-being, and Quality of Life Among Individuals on the Autism Spectrum. *Pediatrics* **141**, S362–S368 (2018).

17. Weitlauf, A. S., Gotham, K. O., Vehorn, A. C. & Warren, Z. E. Brief Report: DSM-5 'Levels of Support:' A Comment on Discrepant Conceptualizations of Severity in ASD. *J. Autism Dev. Disord.* **44**, 471–476 (2014).

18. Mouga, S. *et al.* Intellectual Profiles in the Autism Spectrum and Other Neurodevelopmental Disorders. *J. Autism Dev. Disord.* **46**, 2940–2955 (2016).

19. American Psychiatric Association & DSM-5 Task Force. *Diagnostic and Statistical Manual of Mental Disorders: DSM-5* (American Psychiatric Association, 2013).

20. Baird, G., Douglas, H. R., Director, A. & Murphy, M. S. Recognising and Diagnosing Autism in Children and Young People: Summary of NICE Guidance. *BMJ* **343** (2011).

21. Russell, A. E., Ford, T. & Russell, G. Barriers and Predictors of Medication Use for Childhood ADHD: Findings from a UK Population-representative Cohort. *Soc. Psychiatry Psychiatr. Epidemiol.* **54**, 1555–1564 (2019).

22. Foucault, M. *Archaeology of Knowledge* (Routledge, 2002).

23. Russell, G. & Norwich, B. Dilemmas, Diagnosis and De-stigmatization: Parental Perspectives on the Diagnosis of Autism Spectrum Disorders. *Clin. Child Psychol. Psychiatry* **17**, 229–245 (2012).

24. Eyal, G., Hart, B., Onculer, E., Neta, O. & Rossi, N. *The Autism Matrix* (Polity, 2010).

25. Waltz, M. *Autism: A Social and Medical History* (Palgrave Macmillan, 2013).

26. Frances, A. *Saving Normal: An Insider's Revolt Against Out-of-Control Psychiatric Diagnosis, DSM-5, Big Pharma, and the Medicalization of Ordinary Life* (HarperCollins, 2014).

27. Hacking, I. The Looping Effects of Human Kinds. In *Causal Cognition* (eds. Sperber, D., Premack, D. & Premack, A. J.) (Oxford University Press, 1996). doi:10.1093/acprof:oso/9780198524021.001.0001.

28. Hacking, I. Making Up People. *London Review of Books* 23–26 (2006).

29. Becker, H. S. *Outsiders; Studies in the Sociology of Deviance* (Free Press of Glencoe, 1963).

30. Merton, R. K. The Self-Fulfilling Prophecy. *Antioch Rev.* **8**, 193–210 (1948).

31. Jussim, L. Self-Fulfilling Prophecies: A Theoretical and Integrative Review. *Psychol. Rev.* **93**, 429–445 (1986).

32. Haslam, N. Looping Effects and the Expanding Concept of Mental Disorder. *Off. J. Ital. Soc. Psychopathol.* **22**, 4–9 (2016).

33. Tekin, Ş. The Missing Self in Hacking's Looping Effects. In *Classifying Psychopathology: Mental Kinds and Natural Kinds* (eds. Kincaid, H. & Sullivan, J. A.) 227–256 (MIT Press, 2014).

34. Hacking, I. *Proceedings of the British Academy, Volume 151, 2006 Lectures* (British Academy, 2007).

35. Loomes, R., Hull, L. & Mandy, W. P. L. What is the Male-to-Female Ratio in Autism Spectrum Disorder? A Systematic Review and Meta-Analysis. *J. Am. Acad. Child Adolesc. Psychiatry* **56**, 466–474 (2017).

36. Russell, G. *et al.* Selection Bias on Intellectual Ability in Autism Research: A Cross-sectional Review and Meta-analysis. *Mol. Autism* **10**, 9 (2019).

37. Aronowitz, R. A. When do Symptoms Become a Disease? *Ann. Intern. Med.* **134**, 803–808 (2001).

38. Williams, D. *Nobody Nowhere: The Extraordinary Autobiography of an Autistic* (Avon, 1994).

39. Grandin, T. & Scariano, M. M. *Emergence: Labeled Autistic* (Warner Books, 1996).

40. Sacks, O. W. *An Anthropologist on Mars: Seven Paradoxical Tales* (Knopf, 1995).

41. Hacking, I. Autistic Autobiography. *Philos. Trans. R. Soc. Lond. B. Biol. Sci.* **364**, 1467–1473 (2009).

4   Adults

The time trend

Our 2020 analysis of time trend data covered nine million patients registered in English general practitioner (GP) practices between 1998 and 2018.[1] We compared the trends in diagnosis we derived for pre-school children, primary age children, adolescents and adults. Figure 4.1 illustrates the relative *pace* of increase of diagnosis in adults compared to other groups, showing how the rate of increase in new autism diagnoses was most rapid in adults. Note that, in Figure 4.1, the baseline in 1998 is held at the same level for all four groups, although far more children and adolescents were diagnosed each year than adults. But the graph well illustrates how the rate of increase in diagnosis was greater for adults than other groups.

As already noted, In the first and second editions of the *Diagnostic and Statistical Manual of Mental Disorders* (DSM I and II), autism was a sub-type of childhood schizophrenia; it became an independent condition, infantile autism, in DSM III, published in 1980. As the name implied, autism was then exclusively a diagnosis of childhood. DSM-III-R, which came out in in 1987, dropped the requirement that onset should happen before the child was 30 months old, and in 1994, DSM-IV categorised autism as a spectrum. Adult autism diagnosis is therefore a relatively new concept and practice.

Diagnostic services

In the UK, The Autism Act (2009) made it a statutory requirement for every local authority to provide access to diagnosis for adults, with costs provided by central government, leading to the creation of a national network of adult assessment services in England in the 2010s.[2] The Autism Act was drafted by a coalition of UK autism charities, led by the National Autistic Society[3] and supported by Cheryl Gillan, a Conservative Member of Parliament.

The Autism Act has a place in history as the first disability-specific Act of Parliament in the UK. There is no attention deficit hyperactivity disorder (ADHD) act, no cerebral palsy act, no dementia act. Autism seems to be a particular site of mobilisation, unlike, for example, ADHD. This is partly because

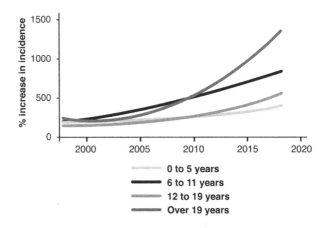

Figure 4.1 Time trend in incidence of new cases in England by age band in primary care data.

of autism's long history of professional and parental waves of advocacy (see Introduction, Figure 2, and multiple texts[4-7]) which created an infrastructure of well-established, well-organised charities and advocacy organisations. A cynic might suggest because there is a well established drug treatment for ADHD it is in the interests of the pharmacological industry to locate ADHD within a medical framework (see Sergio Sismondo's seering account of the ghost management of resistance and advocacy by the pharma industry).[8]

The emphasis of autism lobbying at that time was on the area of least-met need: adulthood. In 2009, very few local authorities in England had adult diagnosis services. By spring 2019 almost all (93%) did.[9] This reflects Roy Richard Grinker's point that rising prevalence estimates inevitably follow an increase in services, with diagnostic (and possibly therapeutic) service availability influencing rates of diagnosis.[10] Jennie Hayes, while researching for her PhD in the *Exploring Diagnosis* team, studied the practice of diagnosing adults in the network of adult autism assessment services, as well as examining the process of autism diagnosis in child services. The network of adult autism assessment centres was distinguished by being founded with the specific task of assessing adults for autism diagnoses.[3] Many adults have come forward for referral since 2010; waiting lists are long, up to four years in some places.[11]

Hayes's work, which analysed discussions in multi-disciplinary diagnostic teams, raised the question of whether the institutional requirements and practices of adult diagnostic services, although founded on the neutral premise of meeting a need, inadvertently co-constituted a growing demand for adult autism diagnosis. The presence of adult assessment services gave oxygen to *the idea* of a new category of autistic adults. The new network of services, together with culturally available materials such as autie-biography, fictional accounts, neurodiversity and so on (Figure 4.2), means adults (and

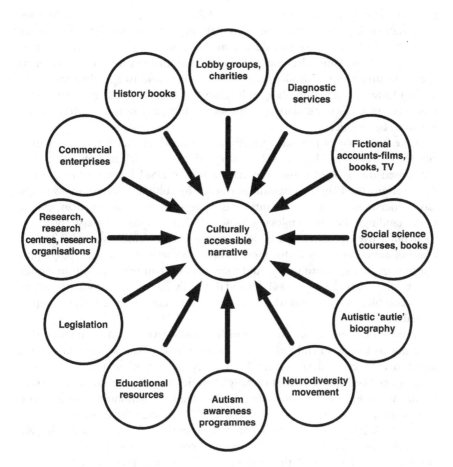

Figure 4.2 Areas where there has been a rise in activity centred on autism as a diagnostic category.

the parents of adults living in the parental home) are now far more likely to consider an autism diagnosis as a *possibility* for explaining their, or their offspring's, experience.

'Autie-biographers'[12–15] are adults with autism who have written about what autism looks like. Their texts have become prototypical accounts of experience on the spectrum. In the UK, we heard that many adults who come to clinic directly cite such stories when seeking an autism diagnosis. UK adults related in particular to the autobiographical accounts of two successful self-proclaimed autistic people: Greta Thunberg[15] and Chris Packham.[16] Packham (who co-incidentally I briefly worked with in a previous life at the BBC's Natural History Unit) is a hugely talented naturalist and presenter, may line up clothes in his wardrobe, yet manages to sustain multiple complex social relationships at work, has a long-term relationship and has been able to nurture his step child into a co-presenting opportunity, is gifted with language, having been highly articulate for many years as a forthright spokesperson on the loss of biodiversity, during a very public and altogether stellar career. These qualities – absolute autonomy, ability to manage complex relationships, extreme fluency in the spoken word – are very far from autism pre-1990. Autism has come a long way. Identifying with autie-biographers like Packham prompts self-identification which may lead to a medical diagnosis, as Tom Lister noted.[17] Autie-biographies help provide the language to style what it is to be autistic, a vocabulary that, for some adults, begins to constitute what it means to be autistic.

Autie-biography is just one of many areas of activity that have made autism culturally accessible (Figure 4.2). Many adults who self-identify as autistic recognised the signs of autism not via the official DSM-5 criteria but through the de-stigmatised lay understandings offered by culturally accessible resources. Lay understandings of what autism is appear to be broader than clinical understandings. People employing biosocial identities do not passively accept them but actively construct the biology on which their identity is based.[18] The net effect of autie-biography is that more people who relate to the autie-biographer opt into the autism community. And they too can then tell their autism stories. Twenty-five years ago, this possibility did not really exist or at least was not culturally accessible; ten years ago, there was no infrastructure (in the UK) to support its realisation.

As noted earlier, an autism diagnosis is usually given to adults because they were not picked up in childhood. Autistic people who have severe neurological impairments, severe developmental delay, are non-verbal or minimally verbal and/or need constant care are normally identified in early life. Adults who come to diagnostic services are most often in the 'higher-functioning' group of autistic people, often with less glaring needs.[19-24] The earlier the diagnosis is made, the more likely an autistic person is to have cognitive and severe autistic impairment, and later diagnoses are more likely to come from the 'threshold' region (Figure 3.1). Members of the group identified in adulthood were 'missed' as children partly because their differences were less obvious and partly because, with time, autism thresholds have crept left in the figure. As adults, the group has been encompassed as diagnosable, whereas when they were children, years ago, they may not have qualified. This is not to say such adults do not struggle with everyday life and face challenges. Some studies suggest adults with higher intellect are more likely to suffer from mental health issues, such as depression, than people with lower[25] perhaps because of a greater self-awareness and consciousness of a discrepancy between their high intellect and ability to achieve success in relationships and at work.[26] Autism severity has been associated with *fewer* bouts of anxiety/depression, lower IQ and smaller number of reciprocal friendships.[27]

The group identified at adulthood is formed of people who have managed school life without a diagnosis of autism. As with the transition to secondary school, the transition to fulfil society's expectation of an independent adult life, and associated decrease in support, may prompt the need for diagnosis as they or their family seek additional services and support. The adult world is simply harder to negotiate; workplaces may lack the support offered by the educational system and families may be unable to provide housing. Adult diagnosis can provide access to services but, more commonly, the adult services in our studies provided diagnosis but not additional services. Nonetheless, many, and perhaps most, adults and their parents found their newly minted autism diagnosis a useful explanatory model for a lifetime of difference: 'I didn't fit in'; 'there was something a bit different about my behaviour'; 'I had something wrong with me'; 'I can always say "Sorry, I have got Asperger syndrome" … the excuse if you like but excuse is not a very good word … the reason … the explanation'.[28]

Hayes's studies of diagnostic services underlined how medical practices, new technologies or new infrastructure create, as well as report on, phenomena, underlining a point made beautifully by Annemarie Mol.[29] Therefore the practice of diagnosing autism cannot be separated from the ontological question of what autism is. As Astrid Schrader puts it, what we know cannot be separated from the *way* that we know it.[30] Autism is an object of knowledge – it is what we know – but it is an object partly delineated by the process of knowing it. This is not in itself problematic but claims that practice, technology or infrastructure are simply the neutral processes of identification that have no impact on the phenomena of interest are unfounded. Autism is rendered an object *through the process of* its identification by health care professionals.[31] Hayes goes on to discuss how clinicians involved in diagnostic decisions were constrained and informed by institutional demands. Adult diagnostic services exist solely to confer (or not) an autism diagnosis, so complex behaviours were inevitably reduced to a yes/no decision, with a cut-off for diagnosis necessarily imposed somewhere in the broad autism phenotype; giving a diagnosis was metaphorically 'drawing a line in the sand', as one clinician pointed out.[31]

To be clear, the adults who came to the services *all* had autistic traits but the question of whether they did or did not have autism was less clear. Hayes collected fascinating data, some of which (at the time of writing) she continues to work on as part of a fellowship.[32] Her data reveal clinicians are in a position of authority – people who, through training and experience, expressed as their 'feel' for autism, can decide who has and who does not have autism. What autism looked like, who could 'sense' it and what it signified to the patient were points of discussion in clinicians' discussion about diagnosis.[33] The strength of the autism 'signal' is an important factor in determining diagnostic outcome but deciding exactly what that signal is returns us to the question of 'what is autism?' For clinicians, this seemed to be negotiable, perhaps due to the uncertainty inherent in autism's heterogeneity, its diverse presentation and its aetiological variation – what Gregory Hollin refers to as autism's 'ontological indeterminacy'.[34]

None of this is to suggest that troubling behaviours – 'symptoms' in medical parlance – are not 'real' but rather that it is nigh-on impossible to disentangle the assessment process: the ways clinicians determine the diagnostic story. The processes through which diagnostic stories are constructed from disparate sources of evidence have been extensively researched by other medical sociologists, including Joanna Latimer,[35] who writes about conferring a diagnosis in her ethnographic study of genetic clinics covering dysmorphology. Other sociological scholars show how clinicians give the impression they are discussing something objective, something 'out there', but, in their discussion of the results of diagnostic tests, testimony and evidence, become the central narrators of diagnostic stories through structured talk and formal spaces.[36]

Autism in Adulthood, the first academic journal specific to adults with autism, was founded in 2018. Its existence shows autism in adulthood now has a strong research, as well as diagnostic focus. The flow of knowledge and attention toward the topic of autism in adulthood boosts the processes of self-identification and lay diagnosis by and of adults. Adults diagnosed with autism often have a strong autistic identity and many in Europe (particularly the UK), and North America (particularly the USA), are self-advocates and have mobilised around the category.

Reasons for mobilisation: the motive

Millions of dollars in funding and investment have been raised on the back of the tragedy narrative of autism. The 2007 Starbucks Coffee Cups and first-wave activism often positioned autism as thoroughly bad, something to be eliminated or cured, a tragedy. The Coffee Cup warning was written by a representative of *Autism Speaks*, a bastion of pro-cure parent activists, who used biological causation of autism to deflect from the earlier, damaging, mother blame theories.

Aligned to the Coffee Cup's dire warnings, the diagnosis of autism as a disorder automatically positions people with autism as people who have something wrong with them. The current definitions of autism spectrum disorder specify a range of behavioural 'deficits'. DSM-5 describes the behavioural traits that constitute the core *symptoms* of autism as 'persistent *deficits* in social communication and social interaction across multiple contexts' and 'restricted, repetitive patterns of behaviour, interests or activities', which may include '*hyper-* or *hypo*-sensitivity or *unusual* interest in sensory aspects of the environment'. Social deficits are primary, including '*deficits* in social-emotional reciprocity', which include '*failure* of normal back-and-forth conversation', '*reduced* sharing of interests, emotions or affect', '*poorly* integrated verbal or non-verbal communication', '*failure* to initiate or respond to social interactions', '*lack of* facial expressions', '*deficits* in developing, maintaining and understanding relationships', '*difficulties* adjusting behaviour' and '*absence of* interest in peers' (my italics).[37, 38]

Thus, the definitive medical text basically describes the condition as a collection of deficits, inevitably damning the person with autism as having something fundamentally amiss: 'You've been officially declared to be this awful dud', as one of the participants in our short film series put it.[39] Autism, as cast in these autism-as-tragedy texts, has traditionally been, a highly stigmatised identity.[40–42] Stigma, as a sociological concept, was developed by Erving Goffman in his pioneering book *Stigma: Notes on the Management of a Spoiled Identity*.[43] Today, both medical and sociological literatures are rife with studies of stigma and how to combat it. Bruce Link and Jo Phelan describe a trade-off between treatment benefits of a diagnosis and effects of stigma, concluding that diagnostic labelling can of itself exert an independent effect on the rejecting responses of the public.[44]

In our study of the accounts of adults with an autism diagnosis we heard how autistic adults experienced autism not as a separate phenomenon but as a core part of their personality.[45] To hear messages reinforcing what they regarded as their core selves as entirely deficient, broken, damaged and disordered, a condition that should inspire fear and panic, is not helpful. Such messages may be internalised and damage self-esteem.[46] Able autistic adults have been, and have felt, heavily discriminated against in very tangible social and economic ways, as well as in interpersonal interaction. Such messages may instead inspire; this group has been *motivated* to stage a mobilised fight-back and reclaim the autistic identity as their own, casting it in a much more positive light – a process of resistance predicted by social identity theory.[47]

Reasons for mobilisation: the means

Since the 1990s, many autistic adults have had not only the motivation but also the *means* to mobilise. These are adults with the ability to use a computer and the Internet has enabled them to meet and rally in virtual spaces.[48] Autistic adults often have difficulties with face-to-face interaction but their fluency in on-line spaces has been well documented.[48] The impact of the Internet is described by Judy Singer, a sociologist 'somewhere on the autistic spectrum',[49] as being akin to the impact of sign language among the deaf.[50]

As noted, the group presenting to adult services is likely to have, on average, a higher IQ and lower support needs than those diagnosed in young childhood.[19-24] Alongside them is now the group of children who became eligible for an autism diagnosis in the 1990s some now grown up into able, computer-literate adults, even as they faced challenges. Some of them are highly fluent in the visual world and have no intellectual impairment. The net result is a growing cohort of creative and intelligent Internet-using adults with an autism diagnosis.

In tandem with the growing use of the Internet as a communication tool, the late 1990s saw a rise in identity-based politics, such as transgender activism, mad pride and survivor movements. Another parallel trend was the growth in the *neuro-centrist* discourse (the tendency to explain people's behaviour in terms of the biology or anatomy of their brains).[51] Singer adopted the neuro-term to describe *neurodiversity*, to her a sub-set of biodiversity, in 1998.[49]

The parallels between the re-defining of autistic identity through neurodiversity and other health-based movements redefining theirs is a topic I have looked at elsewhere with Erica Dyck, a historian of mental health and medicine.[52] By the early 2000s, disability rights, anti-psychiatry and social and medical models were well established and the political, technological and medical conditions were ripe for them to be adapted by a cohort of able autistic adults alienated by descriptions of themselves as broken. The confluence of circumstances enabled the autistic rights and neurodiversity movements to flourish: autistic adults had the numbers, the means (access to Internet-enabled computers), the motivation (as a group they are discriminated against) and the intellectual ability to come together in virtual spaces to change the landscape of autism.

Autistic activism and the neurodiversity movement

One way the landscape has changed is its encompassing of *autism-as-identity* or autistic identity, which is slowly making inroads into the medical bastions and troubling the notion of *autism-as-disorder*. Activists want autistic people to be identified but in an alternative, more holistic and realistic classification that places increasing emphasis on patient expertise and lived experience.[53] This is a core concept in medical sociology; theorists such as Donna Haraway have been instrumental in replacing old ideas such as 'non-compliance' and physicians bending patients to their will with the concept that everyone's 'lay knowledge' is valued and contextual.[54] People's beliefs about their health and identity are, in part, representations of the culture and society in which they live. Autism, and the way it is understood by different actors, becomes a social mirror that reflects our world.

The difficulty lies in reconciling the various forms of expertise. Kapp and colleagues have described the expertise of adults who have lived experience of autism.[55] Clearly, lay expertise is different from lived expertise, which differs from professional expertise, although a person can have all three. There is a power imbalance, with the lay forms of expertise being treated as inferior to the professional forms. For this reason, in the *Exploring Diagnosis* volume edited by Kapp,[56] we foregrounded autistic voices. In the face of constructive criticism from Ari Ne'eman, I dropped off the editorial team, to allow solely autistic editorship and control. Although giving up my place was at the time painful, stepping back was undoubtedly for the best. The autistic voices were uninterrupted, able to tell their own story. And I was free to develop my idea for this book. It was a lesson that releasing control is sometimes the best contribution you can make.

Lay or lived expertise, according to Beck,[57] has a distinct role in setting the research question of interest. In theory the lay positions are embodied by elected agents in government, while the role of the professional expert is to advise on methods and sometimes implement the methods of obtaining these goals. The aim of apportioning different roles to distinct forms of expertise is to enjoy the advantages of division of labour while treating each other as equals, as Thomas Christiano argues in his work on democracy.[58] The mobilisation of autistic adults in the neurodiversity movement is an example of how lay knowledge is influencing the professional medical agenda. As the response to Covid-19 has shown, there is sometimes a need to defer to scientific experts but also to understand and critique all forms of expertise and demand transparency in how decisions are shaped. Otherwise, risk and resistance narratives, both scientific and lay, can either be used to justify power grabs or become entrenched.

Does a person with lived experience have more authority than other types of people? Their experience is valid and important, certainly. But people with lived experience are sometimes the most enthusiastic advocates of abhorrent practices. For example, 120 million girls and women have been subject to female genital mutilation (FGM) in Africa, Asia and the Middle East.[59] FGM involves cutting out the external female genitalia of girls in infancy, childhood or adolescence, resulting in multiple and horrific short- and long-term health issues, including shock, bleeding, severe pain, pain during intercourse, menstrual problems, chronic infection, increased risk of problems in childbirth and death.[60] In some regions, FGM is promoted and advocated by grandmothers who have themselves undergone this vicious and oppressive practice, that is, the people with lived experience. In the context of their lives, grandmothers understand that the mutilation may protect their granddaughters from early or unplanned pregnancy, ensures premarital virginity and marital fidelity and increases marriageability.[61] Lived experience does not *necessarily* lead to progressive resistance; it can also uphold oppressive and damaging norms. Such stories should be heard, and are valid. But they are not necessarily to be agreed with.

Kapp's edited volume tells the stories of some of the main autistic players in the neurodiversity movement. The contributors include Martijn Dekker, who created InLv, the first autistic-run Internet forum, the late Mel Baggs, who inspired many with their video blog *In My Language*,[62] a commentary on personhood and what it means to be excluded, and Ari Ne'eman, who, as president of the Autistic Self Advocacy Network (ASAN) in 2012, was the primary driver in the lobbying of the DSM-5 neurodevelopmental working group.[53]

The history of autistic activism and the neurodiversity movement has been covered extensively, so I will not dwell on it.[7, 8, 63–65] However, two pieces of writing are worth mentioning: the essays by the autistic pioneer, Jim Sinclair: 'Don't Mourn for Us' written in 1992–1993[64] and 'Why I Dislike "Person First" Language', written in 1999.[65] Both were republished in 2012–2013. The influence of these twin works has reverberated down the years. 'Don't Mourn for Us' asked parents to accept children with autism, not treat them as a tragedy; to enter the child's world, not normalise and force them into unwanted change.[64] In 'Why I Dislike "Person First" Language' Sinclair expressed similar sentiments to the participants in our research: autism was an important aspect of their sense of self.[65]

Traditionally, 'autistic' was thought to be stigmatising as a derogatory term because it implied that the person *was* a problem, rather than *had* a problem. Sinclair's argument in support of person-first language (e.g. 'autistic adult') is that autism was an integral part of who he was, with both challenges and strengths, not an aspect that he cared to shed or recover from. 'Autistic' is equivalent to any other characteristic of a person, such as their sex, gender or sexuality. Describing a 'person with autism' is equivalent to saying 'person with femaleness' or 'person with gayness' and implies that the gayness or femaleness or autism can be removed. This, Sinclair argued, cannot be done and nor should one attempt to do so. 'Cancerous person' would never be used; cancer is a life-threatening disease, whereas autism is not, and should not be conceived as one.

Sinclair was pioneering in his descriptions of being autistic, re-casting autism as an identity and, by re-framing autism in an affirmative way, hitting a nerve. All the adult autistic activists I have met use the term 'autistic' to describe themselves. While many older psychiatry journals, such as the *Journal of Child Psychology and Psychiatry*, only allow authors to use the descriptor 'person with autism', progressive journals such as *Autism* allow the use of both terms, and in some newer journals, such as *Autism in Adulthood*, the use of 'autistic' is mandatory. In this book I use both, which may date the text.

The Internet means adults with autism can communicate over wide geographical spaces and share news. Autism was the banner around which positive collective identities were asserted and from which the identity politics of the neurodiversity movement emerged.[66-71] 'Neurodiversity' implies that neurological difference is an inherent and valuable part of human variation, not a pathology. The neurodiversity movement advocates de-medicalisation, as its intention is to class deviant (neurodivergent) behaviour as a normal human framework, not a diagnosable condition. However, at the same time, many of the autistic activists who founded the neurodiversity movement advocate for increased access to diagnosis, as diagnosis brings services, accommodations, identity and rights.

Kapp and I conducted an analysis of autistic adults' responses to the question 'What is neurodiversity, in your own words?', originally posed in a study Kapp co-led with Kristen Gillespie Lynch.[55] We found that the data largely mapped on to definitions autistic adults in the movement have given. For example, Nick Walker described the neurodiversity movement as encompassing both human biological differences in cognition, brains and genes, while also serving as an activist device for change, promoting the acceptance and inclusion of autistic and other neurodivergent people.[72]

Collective identity based on shared biological difference is arguably a form of Paul Rabinow's 'biosociality'[73] or Nikolas Rose and Carlos Novas's 'biological citizenship'.[74] These ideas incorporate neurodivergent and autistic as an identity for adults who either have a diagnosis or self-identify, a phenomenon described at length by autistic activists and others.[75-78] Francisco Ortega has called the business of emphasising autism as *brain*-based the practice of 'cerebralising' or 'neurologisation', understanding autism (or any condition) in terms of differences in brain 'wiring' or structure.[79] An over-emphasis on a brain-based model tends to de-emphasise developmental and social influences. I covered this, and other major critiques of the neurodiversity movement, in a chapter for Kapp's collection.[80] Some have argued that the higher-functioning autistic men who have dominated the neurodiversity movement represent those who least need help.[80] Focusing attention on the brain can also underplay other physiological issues; epilepsy is clearly neurological but co-morbidities such as gastro-intestinal problems, endocrine, metabolic and motor difficulties are de-emphasised. One of the criticisms of the movement is that it pays rather little attention to the problems arising from these co-occurring 'specifiers' (DSM-5) and it also leads to confusion when some (parent) advocates call for treatments for autism; often they want to treat the specifiers/co-morbidities. These semantic problems can lead to category errors and mutual suspicion between parent advocates and autistic adults.

Critiques notwithstanding, the neurodiversity movement broadly aims to counter discrimination, stigmatisation and prejudice. People aligned to the movement have put forward several broad principles:

1. Use identity-first language ('dyslexic', not 'person with dyslexia'). Thus, the neuro-attribute is re-designated as part of personhood/identity, not framed as disease.
2. Autism, ADHD and dyslexia and other neurodevelopmental conditions are best thought of as disabilities, not disorders.
3. Acknowledge the advantages that autism and other neuro-disabilities may bring: that having extreme neurodivergence may contribute to society in unexpected and positive ways and that it is therefore important to retain it in the gene pool, affirming the validity of impairment, in line with the affirmative model of disability.
4. Being autistic, having ADHD, diagnosed or not, is a valid way to be and neurodivergent people should be included and accepted.
5. The principle of self-determination, encapsulated in the slogan 'Nothing about us without us'.[81] Autistic and other neurodivergent people claim expertise by dint of their lived experience. Advocates argue their point of view must be heard as valid.
6. Children with neuro-disabilities are not problems to be fixed but people to be understood and supported in a mutually respectful relationship.[63]
7. The movement is broadly anti-cure but neurodivergent people should have the right to various supports, including but not limited to facilitated communication, support at school, accommodations and being protected, by the law, from discrimination.[82] Autistic and other neurodivergent people require respect for their personal integrity, support for special talents and assistance with tasks they find difficult.[63]

Thus, the movement places the autism spectrum within the human spectrum, alongside other forms of diversity, including race, gender, sexuality and their accompanying discourses of rights, freedoms and self-determination.[63] Neurodiversity has simultaneously opposed, adopted and co-opted aspects of the biomedical discourse, using a primarily brain-based understanding. ASAN has advocated for broadened diagnosis while at the same time opposing a disease- and solely deficit-based concept of autism. Both activist (autistic-as-identity) and medical (autism-as-disorder) narratives seem to reify autism in different ways. Autistic rights activists use the diagnostic category to rally and to underpin rights-based discourse. Their strong identity has led some autistics to envisage a separatist autistic state, as Joseph Redford wrote in a personal communication, a fascinating story I was sadly unable to convince the editors to include in the resulting volume.

One way the movement shaped medical knowledge about autism was ASAN's lobbying of the neurodevelopmental work group that prepared the DSM-5 criteria for autism.[53] This alliance was a symbiotic partnership that led to tangible changes in the final DSM-5 text. Although one might not think them natural bedfellows, both parties benefitted. The lived experiential expertise of ASAN lent credibility to and legitimised the efforts of the neurodevelopmental work group in the eyes of the autism community, benefitting the scientists. At the same time, the work group provided a successful platform from which autistic activists could lobby for changes to the diagnostic criteria. Kapp acted as ASAN's scientific officer, reviewing autism literature while researching for a PhD at UCLA and using the language of science. In this way ASAN co-opted the scientific discourse and became respected experts, able to converse fluently with the scientists involved. Their experience is reminiscent of the AIDS activists of the mid-1980s, who campaigned to be allowed to participate in drug trials.[83] Credibility tactics emerged, in which activist patients familiarised themselves with the language of science and employed scientific discourse, leading to a successful conclusion.

For some, neurodiversity has a broad definition, encompassing autism, dyslexia, dyspraxia, dyscalculia, dysgraphia, Tourette's syndrome, anxiety disorders, obsessive compulsive disorder, ADHD, cerebral palsy, dementia and depression, although some operationalise narrower definitions, covering just the autism spectrum.[84] Singer regards neurodiversity as a subset of biodiversity, in the sense that neurodiversity is as important for a viable culture as biodiversity is for a viable ecosystem.[85] She is sceptical of the categorisation of people (for example, as 'neurodivergent'), arguing this will stigmatise the category and become a way to denote 'the other'. In autism research, 'neurotypical' is often used to describe the dominant 'other' – for example, a control group that does not have autism – although this is inaccurate, as such groups may contain many neurodiverse people. In this context, the word 'allistic', coined by the autism community, is more accurate. Allistic simply means 'not autistic', without the impossibility of 'neurotypical'.

The more progressive term for neurodivergent is perhaps neuro-disability, which nods to the social model of disability.[86] The social model differentiates between a person's impairment and the disabling structures and practices they encounter, which interact to prevent their full participation in society. A person's impairment might be paraplegia but their disablement would be caused by lack of wheelchair access to buildings. Of course, unless one delineates who qualifies as neurodivergent, one can't use it as a marker for delivering rights or providing enhanced access or services. Whether qualification for the group of those who are neurodivergent should be through a medical diagnosis or self-identification is unclear. Who it incorporates may be vague because the neurodiversity movement rose spontaneously, in reaction to what were perceived as oppressive discourses and practices, not via a top-down doctrine.[5]

Despite being problematised, the work of neurodiversity activists has had the net result of reshaping the autism landscape into a more progressive, less stigmatising form. Autism is no longer seen as a withdrawal or inability to interact with the world but, rather, a different kind of contact with it. Manuel Castells's seminal book, *The Power of Identity*, describes a *resistance identity* that challenges the devaluation and stigmatisation of the group that constructs it and seeks the

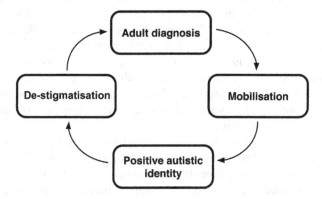

Figure 4.3 The looping effect of mobilisation and de-stigmatisation.

transformation of the overall social structure.[87] Neurodiversity and autistic identity are forms of resistance to the dominant risk and tragedy discourses about
autism. Activists have worked towards more legislation and increased access to
support; many medical, social and cultural resources that de-stigmatise autism
and reframe autism-as-identity have been produced as a result. This is undeni-
ably very good for autistic people and their self-worth and something we can all
applaud. But there is a consequence: looping.

As autism becomes progressively de-stigmatised, so a more positive autistic
identity is shaped. Subsequently, and in tandem, more adults are likely to self-
identify and many (but not all) will self-refer for diagnostic assessment.[17] The
consequence of mobilisation and de-stigmatisation is thus more autism diagnoses. And more autism diagnosis mean more adults acting for de-stigmatisation
(Figure 4.3).

If *self-diagnosis* is the process through which an adult comes to believe they
are autistic, *lay diagnosis* is the process through which someone who is not medically qualified tags someone else with a diagnostic label. As diagnosis is technic-
ally something only a clinician can administer, some consider that lay diagnosis
is an oxymoron, similar to the term *lay expert*.[88] Many autistic adults prefer the
term *self-identification*. Thomas Lister studied these twin diagnostic processes
for autism as part of his PhD research.[17] He found a lay diagnosis is often conferred by a parent, relative or teacher on a child. Some people with autism even
claimed to have a special 'autie-dar' (by analogy with 'gay-dar'); the ability to
spot another person with autism who has not 'come out'. Thus, knowing about
autism renders autism visible in others. And autism-as-a-label is easier both to
assign and own when its connotations become more positive.

There are many interventions that aim to combat stigma. Perhaps the best
way to promote de-stigmatisation of health conditions is to harness the power
of resistance engendered by health-based activist collectives, such as the
neurodiversity movement.[89] Stigma is a relational process emerging from political

forces of dominance and oppression that maintains and creates relations of power and control, as it causes 'some groups to feel devalued and others to feel they are superior in some way'.[89] Many years ago, Pierre Bourdieu argued that the dominated are taught to accept their lot through cultural hegemony, the understanding of social hierarchy.[90] In a culture in which people with autism, ADHD and other conditions have traditionally been devalued and have lower social status, a resistance identity can challenge this narrative through activism. Anti-stigma efforts can be most effective when they support and bolster existing activism and grassroots campaigns.[89]

Since the 1990s, the rise in activity around autism as a diagnostic category for adults has led to both more diagnosis and a surge in mobilised activity in the autism rights and neurodiversity movements. It is worth remembering that autism in adulthood is a new, and escalating, concept. Adults have always had the type of behaviours that we now understand to lie on the autism spectrum but understanding autism as a diagnostic option for adults is relatively new. The founding of a network of services to diagnose adults and the mobilisation of adult autistic advocates in the neurodiversity movement who claim a progressive autistic identity have created a more de-stigmatised and culturally accessible narrative about adult autism that has fuelled autism's rise.

References

1. Russell, G. *et al.* Time Trends in Autism Diagnosis Over 20 Years: A UK Population-based Cohort Study (in preparation) (2020).
2. Department of Health. Statutory Guidance for Local Authorities and NHS Organisations to Support Implementation of the Adult Autism Strategy. 66. www.gov.uk/government/publications/adult-autism-strategy-statutory-guidance (2015).
3. UK Government. Autism Act 2009. www.legislation.gov.uk/ukpga/2009/15/contents (2009).
4. Evans, B. *The Metamorphosis of Autism: A History of Child Development in Britain* (Manchester University Press, 2017).
5. Eyal, G., Hart, B., Onculer, E., Neta, O. & Rossi, N. *The Autism Matrix* (Polity, 2010).
6. Silverman, C. *Understanding Autism: Parents, Doctors, and the History of a Disorder* (Princeton University Press, 2011).
7. Silberman, S. *Neurotribes: The Legacy of Autism and How to Think Smarter About People Who Think Differently* (Allen & Unwin, 2015).
8. Sismondo, S. *Ghost-managed Medicine: Big Pharma's Invisible Hands.* (Mattering Press, 2018).
9. National Autistic Society. Autism Strategy Overview www.autism.org.uk/about/strategy/overview.aspx (2019).
10. Grinker, R. R. *Unstrange Minds: Remapping the World of Autism* (Basic Books, 2008).
11. National Autistic Society. Autism Diagnosis Postcode Lottery Exposed (18 July 2018). www.autism.org.uk/get-involved/media-centre/news/2018-07-18-autism-diagnosis-postcode-lottery-exposed.aspx (2018).
12. Williams, D. *Nobody Nowhere: The Extraordinary Autobiography of an Autistic* (Avon, 1994).
13. Grandin, T. & Scariano, M. M. *Emergence: Labeled Autistic* (Warner Books, 1996).

14. Tammet, D. *Born on a Blue Day: Inside the Extraordinary Mind of an Autistic Savant* (Free Press, 2007).
15. The Guardian. Greta Thunberg Responds to Asperger's Critics: 'It's a Superpower'. www.theguardian.com/environment/2019/sep/02/greta-thunberg-responds-to-aspergers-critics-its-a-superpower (2019).
16. Packham, C. *Fingers in the Sparkle Jar: A Memoir* (Ebury Press, 2017).
17. Lister, T. *What's in a Label? An Exploration of How People Acquire the Label 'Autistic' in Adulthood and the Consequences of Doing So* (University of Exeter, 2020).
18. Wehling, P. The 'Technoscientization' of Medicine and its Limits: Technoscientific Identities, Biosocialities, and Rare Disease Patient Organizations. *Poiesis Prax.* **8**, 67–82 (2011).
19. Brett, D., Warnell, F., McConachie, H. & Parr, J. R. Factors Affecting Age at ASD Diagnosis in UK: No Evidence that Diagnosis Age has Decreased Between 2004 and 2014. *J. Autism Dev. Disord.* **46**, 1974–1984 (2016).
20. Fountain, C., King, M. D. & Bearman, P. S. Age of Diagnosis for Autism: Individual and Community Factors Across 10 Birth Cohorts. *J. Epidemiol. Community Health* **65**, 503–510 (2011).
21. Mandell, D. S., Novak, M. M. & Zubritsky, C. D. Factors Associated with Age of Diagnosis Among Children with Autism Spectrum Disorders. *Pediatrics* **116**, 1480–1486 (2005).
22. Shattuck, P. T. *et al.* Timing of Identification Among Children with an Autism Spectrum Disorder: Findings from a Population-based Surveillance Study. *J. Am. Acad. Child Adolesc. Psychiatry* **48**, 474–483 (2009).
23. Williams, E., Thomas, K., Sidebotham, H. & Emond, A. Prevalence and Characteristics of Autistic Spectrum Disorders in the ALSPAC Cohort. *Dev. Med. Child Neurol.* **50**, 672–677 (2008).
24. Zwaigenbaum, L. *et al.* Developmental Functioning and Symptom Severity Influence Age of Diagnosis in Canadian Preschool Children with Autism. *Paediatr. Child Health* **24**, e57–e65 (2019).
25. Sterling, L., Dawson, G., Estes, A. & Greenson, J. Characteristics Associated with Presence of Depressive Symptoms in Adults with Autism Spectrum Disorder. *J. Autism Dev. Disord.* **38**, 1011–1018 (2008).
26. Kapp, S. K. Social Support, Well-being, and Quality of Life Among Individuals on the Autism Spectrum. *Pediatrics* **141**, S362–S368 (2018).
27. Mazurek, M. O. & Kanne, S. M. Friendship and Internalizing Symptoms Among Children and Adolescents with ASD. *J. Autism Dev. Disord.* **40**, 1512–1520 (2010).
28. Punshon, C., Skirrow, P. & Murphy, G. The Not Guilty Verdict: Psychological Reactions to a Diagnosis of Asperger Syndrome in Adulthood. *Autism Int. J. Res. Pract.* **13**, 265–283 (2009).
29. Mol, A. *The Body Multiple: Ontology in Medical Practice* (Duke University Press, 2003).
30. Schrader, A. Responding to *Pfiesteria piscicida* (the Fish Killer): Phantomatic Ontologies, Indeterminacy, and Responsibility in Toxic Microbiology. *Soc. Stud. Sci.* **40**, 275–306 (2010).
31. Hayes, J., McCabe, R., Ford, T. & Russell, G. Drawing a Line in the Sand: Affect and Testimony in Autism Assessment Teams in the UK. *Sociol. Health Illn.* **42**, 825–843 (2020).
32. Hayes, J., MacCabe, R., Ford, T. & Russell, G. 'Not at the Diagnosis Point': Dealing with Contradiction in Autism Assessment Teams. *Soc. Sci. Med.* 113462 (2020). doi:10.1016/j.socscimed.2020.113462.

33. Timmermans, S. & Haas, S. Towards a Sociology of Disease. *Sociol. Health Illn.* **30**, 659–676 (2008).

34. Hollin, G. Autistic Heterogeneity: Linking Uncertainties and Indeterminacies. *Sci. Cult.* **26**, 209–231 (2017).

35. Latimer, J. *The Gene, the Clinic, and the Family: Diagnosing Dysmorphology, Reviving Medical Dominance* (Routledge, 2013).

36. Maynard, D. W. & Turowetz, J. J. Doing Testing: How Concrete Competence can Facilitate or Inhibit Performances of Children with Autism Spectrum Disorder. *Qual. Sociol.* **40**, 467–491 (2017).

37. WHO. *International Classification of Diseases, 11th Revision (ICD-11)*. (WHO, 2018). www.who.int/classifications/icd/en/.

38. American Psychiatric Association & DSM-5 Task Force. *Diagnostic and Statistical Manual of Mental Disorders, Fifth Edition* (American Psychiatric Publishing, 2013).

39. Exploring Diagnosis. *The State of Being Different*. (2019). www.youtube.com/watch?v=AGn8OMGLo7Q&t=1s.

40. Farrugia, D. Exploring Stigma: Medical Knowledge and the Stigmatisation of Parents of Children Diagnosed with Autism Spectrum Disorder. *Sociol. Health Illn.* (2009) doi:10.1111/j.1467-9566.2009.01174.x.

41. Gray, D. E. Perceptions of Stigma: The Parents of Autistic Children. *Sociol. Health Illn.* **15**, 102–120 (1993).

42. Russell, G. & Norwich, B. Dilemmas, Diagnosis and De-stigmatization: Parental Perspectives on the Diagnosis of Autism Spectrum Disorders. *Clin. Child Psychol. Psychiatry* **17**, 229–245 (2012).

43. Goffman, E. *Stigma: Notes on the Management of Spoiled Identity* (Touchstone, 1986).

44. Link, B. G. & Phelan, J. C. Stigma and its Public Health Implications. *The Lancet* **367**, 528–529 (2006).

45. Russell, G. *et al.* Mapping the Autistic Advantage from the Accounts of Adults Diagnosed with Autism: A Qualitative Study. *Autism Adulthood* **1**, 124–133 (2019).

46. Milton, D. & Sims, T. How is a Sense of Well-being and Belonging Constructed in the Accounts of Autistic Adults? *Disabil. Soc.* **31**, 520–534 (2016).

47. Major, B. & Crocker, J. Social Stigma and Self-esteem: The Self-protective Properties of Stigma. *Psychol. Rev.* **96**, 608–630 (1989).

48. Davidson, J. Autistic Culture Online: Virtual Communication and Cultural Expression on the Spectrum. *Soc. Cult. Geogr.* **9**, 791–806 (2008).

49. Singer, J. *NeuroDiversity: The Birth of an Idea* (Judy Singer, 2016).

50. Singer, J. 'Why can't you be Normal for Once in Your Life?' From a 'Problem with no Name' to the Emergence of a New Category of Difference (Chapter 7). In *Disability discourse* (eds. Singer, J. & French, S.) vol. Disability, Human Rights, and Society 59–67 (Open University Press, 1999).

51. Satel, S. & Lilienfeld, S. O. *Brainwashed: The Seductive Appeal of Mindless Neuroscience* (Basic Civitas Books, 2013).

52. Dyck, E. & Russell, G. Challenging Psychiatric Classification: Healthy Autistic Diversity, the Neurodiversity Movement. In *Mental Health in Historical Perspective: Healthy Minds in the Twentieth Century* (eds. Taylor, S. J. & Brumby, A.) (Palgrave MacMillan, 2020).

53. Kapp, S. & Ne'eman, A. Lobbying Autism's Diagnostic Revision in the DSM-5. In *Autistic Community and the Neurodiversity Movement – Stories from the Frontline* (Palgrave MacMillan, 2020).

54. Haraway, D. Situated Knowledges: The Science Question in Feminism and the Privilege of Partial Perspective. *Fem. Stud.* **14**, 575–599 (1988).
55. Gillespie-Lynch, K., Kapp, S. K., Brooks, P. J., Pickens, J. & Schwartzman, B. Whose Expertise Is It? Evidence for Autistic Adults as Critical Autism Experts. *Front. Psychol.* **8**, 438 (2017).
56. Kapp, S. K. *Autistic Community and the Neurodiversity Movement: Stories from the Frontline* (Springer Singapore, 2020).
57. Beck, U. *World Risk Society* (Polity Press, 1999).
58. Christiano, T. Democracy. In The Stanford Encyclopedia of Philosophy (ed. Zalta, E. N.) (Metaphysics Research Lab, Stanford University, 2018).
59. Vogt, S., Efferson, C. & Fehr, E. The Risk of Female Genital Cutting in Europe: Comparing Immigrant Attitudes Toward Uncut Girls with Attitudes in a Practicing Country. *SSM – Popul. Health* **3**, 283–293 (2017).
60. WHO. Female genital mutilation. www.who.int/news-room/fact-sheets/detail/female-genital-mutilation (2020).
61. Almroth, L. *et al.* A Community Based Study on the Change of Practice of Female Genital Mutilation in a Sudanese Village. *Int. J. Gynecol. Obstet.* **74**, 179–185 (2001).
62. Baggs, A. *In my Language.* Video blog. www.youtube.com/watch?reload=9&v=JnylM1hI2jc (2007).
63. Waltz, M. *Autism: A Social and Medical History* (Palgrave Macmillan, 2013).
64. Sinclair, J. Don't Mourn for Us. *Auton. Crit. J. Interdiscip. Autism Stud.* **1**, (2012).
65. Sinclair, J. Why I Dislike 'Person First' Language. *Auton. Crit. J. Interdiscip. Autism Stud.* **1** (2013).
66. Baker, D. L. Neurodiversity, Neurological Disability and the Public Sector: Notes on the Autism Spectrum. *Disabil. Soc.* **21**, 15–29 (2006).
67. Brownlow, C. Re-presenting Autism: The Construction of 'NT Syndrome'. *J. Med. Humanit.* **31**, 243–255 (2010).
68. Bumiller, K. Quirky Citizens: Autism, Gender, and Reimagining Disability. *Signs* **33**, 967–991 (2008).
69. Cascio, M. A. Neurodiversity: Autism Pride Among Mothers of Children with Autism Spectrum Disorders. *Intellect. Dev. Disabil.* **50**, 273–283 (2012).
70. Hart, B. Autism Parents and Neurodiversity: Radical Translation, Joint Embodiment and the Prosthetic Environment. *BioSocieties* **9**, 284–303 (2014).
71. Fenton, A. & Krahn, T. Autism, Neurodiversity and Equality Beyond the 'Normal'. *J. Ethics Ment. Health* **2**, 2 (2009).
72. Walker, N. What is Neurodiversity? *Autistic UK* https://autisticuk.org/neurodiversity/ (2014).
73. Rabinow, P. Artificiality and Enlightenment: From Sociobiology to Biosociality. In *Anthropogies of Modernity* (ed. Inda, J. X.) 91–111 (Blackwell Publishing, 1996).
74. Rose, N. & Novas, C. Biological Citizenship. In *Global Assemblages: Technology, Politics, and Ethics as Anthropological Problems* (eds. Ong, A. & Collier, S. J.) 439–463 (Blackwell Publishing, 2005).
75. Sarrett, J. C. & Kapp, S. K. Self-identification and Self-diagnosis in the Autistic Community. In *Disability in American Life* (eds. Heller, T., Parker Harris, S., Gill, C. & Gould, R.) (ABC-CLIO, 2018).
76. Yergeau, M. Occupying Autism: Rhetoric, Involuntarity, and the Meaning of Autistic Lives. In *Occupying Disability: Critical Approaches to Community, Justice, and Decolonizing Disability* (eds. Block, P., Kasnitz, D., Nishida, A. & Pollard, N.) 83–95 (Springer Netherlands, 2016). doi:10.1007/978-94-017-9984-3_6.

77. Lewis, L. F. Exploring the Experience of Self-diagnosis of Autism Spectrum Disorder in Adults. *Arch. Psychiatr. Nurs.* **30**, 575–580 (2016).

78. O'Dell, L., Rosqvist, H. B., Ortega, F., Brownlow, C. & Orsini, M. Critical Autism Studies: Exploring Epistemic Dialogues and Intersections, Challenging Dominant Understandings of Autism. *Disabil. Soc.* **31**, 166–179 (2016).

79. Ortega, F. The Cerebral Subject and the Challenge of Neurodiversity. *BioSocieties* **4**, 425–445 (2009).

80. Russell, G. Critiques of the Neurodiversity Movement. In *Autistic Community and the Neurodiversity Movement: Stories from the Frontline* (ed. Kapp, S. K.) 287–303 (Springer, 2020). doi:10.1007/978-981-13-8437-0_21.

81. Charlton, J. I. *Nothing About Us Without Us: Disability Oppression and Empowerment* (University of California Press, 2000).

82. Broderick, A. A. & Ne'eman, A. Autism as Metaphor: Narrative and Counter-narrative. *Int. J. Incl. Educ.* **12**, 459–476 (2008).

83. Epstein, S. The Construction of Lay Expertise: AIDS Activism and the Forging of Credibility in the Reform of Clinical Trials. *Sci. Technol. Hum. Values* **20**, 408–437 (1995).

84. r/neurodiversity – What 'conditions', 'disorders', or other diagnoses count as neurodivergent? *reddit* www.reddit.com/r/neurodiversity/comments/6u2gcx/what_conditions_disorders_or_other_diagnoses/ (2018).

85. Singer. NeuroDiversity 2.0: What is Neurodiversity? *NeuroDiversity 2.0* https://neurodiversity2.blogspot.com/p/what.html.

86. Oliver, M. *The Politics of Disablement: A Sociological Approach* (Palgrave Macmillan, 1997).

87. Castells, M. *The Power of Identity: The Information Age – Economy, Society, and Culture: 2* (Wiley-Blackwell, 2009).

88. Prior, L. Belief, Knowledge and Expertise: The Emergence of the Lay Expert in Medical Sociology. *Sociol. Health Illn.* **25**, 41–57 (2003).

89. Parker, R. & Aggleton, P. HIV and AIDS-related Stigma and Discrimination: A Conceptual Framework and Implications for Action. *Soc. Sci. Med. 1982* **57**, 13–24 (2003).

90. Bourdieu, P. & Boltanski, L. *La Production de l'idéologie dominante* (Editions Demopolis, 2008).

5 Women on the verge of the autism spectrum

Autism and women

Autism has long been a condition diagnosed primarily in men. A comprehensive review of 43 studies published between 1966 and 2008 found four men with autism to every one woman to be the median ratio.[1] For Asperger's syndrome/disorder (the categories dropped by the most recent revisions to the fifth edition of the *Diagnostic and Statistical Manual of Mental Disorders* (DSM-5) and the 11th edition of the *International Classification of Diseases* (ICD-11)), the gender ratio is thought to be higher: Lorna Wing's famous study estimated 15 men to one woman.[2]

The gender ratio seems to interact with intelligence quotient (IQ) and/or functioning. Most research since the 1990s indicates the male-to-female ratio for adults with autism increases with IQ.[3, 4] An English study found there was no statistically significant difference in the proportion of adult men and women with autism and intellectual disability (ID).[5] By contrast, there were between eight and nine men to every one woman in the group that did not have ID. The study concluded the problem of 'missed' diagnosis is particularly acute for higher-functioning women.

Various reasons for the preponderance of males with autism have been put forward as theories to explain the gender ratio. First, sex-linked genetic differences mean that females are less likely to inherit autistic traits than males.[6] There is also generally greater variation among males, meaning more men at both extremes for a range of traits, including intellectual ability,[7] maths and reading ability[8] and height. Many diagnosable cognitive difficulties are more common in males; for example, specific reading delay, hyperactivity, clumsiness, stammering, ID and Tourette's syndrome.[9] The sex linkage is known as the female protective effect;[10] women have two X chromosomes, meaning the inherited genes work in tandem, whereas men have an XY pair in which the Y chromosomes are unable to modify the effects of the X chromosomes. Most genetic mutations are by nature recessive; for women (XX), this means mutations are only expressed when the same mutation occurs in both copies of the X chromosome. Men (XY) lack this protection, meaning a recessive mutation present in the X chromosome is expressed unconditionally. Hence genetic mutations are expressed more often in men.[11]

However, if the unequal gender ratio in autism is primarily due to the female protective effect, we might expect the ratio of inequality to be greater for people with very low cognitive ability, which is not seen in the data.[3, 4]

A second proposed reason is that infant boys are more susceptible than baby girls to many infections,[12] some of which may be plausible risk factors for autism (see Part II). A third suggestion, the 'extreme male brain' theory of autism,[13] posits autism could partially be caused by the effects of foetal testosterone on brain development.[14] Other early sex-linked hormone exposures could also cause epigenetic change, altering gene expression in male foetuses more often than in female.[15] It is plausible that a combination of these and other explanations contributes to the high male-to-female ratio seen in both autism and other neurodevelopmental conditions.

Since 2010, the four-to-one gender ratio has been questioned, and an autism narrative has developed around 'missed' girls and women; that is, girls and women who miss out on diagnosis because they are under-recognised.[16] Evidence of the missing-ness of women comes from a global systematic review that analysed 54 studies containing data about more than 50,000 participants with autism.[3] This review found that the male-to-female ratio in participants with an autism diagnosis (those reaching clinics) was just over four to one, whereas in population-based studies, the ratio estimates were less, on average around three to one. The conclusion was that there are more women and girls with autism than receive a diagnosis or make it to a clinic. Epidemiological population-based estimates of attention deficit hyperactivity disorder (ADHD) also tend to give a lower gender ratio than estimates based on clinical data[17] and there is a very similar narrative around the missing diagnosis of women in the ADHD literature.[18]

Missing women

At a clinicians' workshop held in London at the end of 2019, I attended a talk entitled *Women and ASD: Missed Diagnosis and Misdiagnosis*, taken from a paper with a similar name.[19] The speaker, a clinical psychologist, posed a question and immediately answered it herself:

'Are women with autism missed?'

'Yes'.

Missing-ness, it is often argued, is important if, through lack of or missed diagnosis, girls and women lose access to crucial services and self-understanding. My PhD work corroborated the 'missed' story: being female was a predictor of lack of autism diagnosis: we found that boys were more likely to receive a diagnosis than girls even when levels of their autistic traits were comparable.[20] We wondered if stereotyping autism as 'male' (perhaps prompted by the 'extreme male brain' theory of autism) might lead to biases in recognition if clinicians, parents and teachers see autism as primarily a 'male' disorder. The male neurodevelopmental stereotype might contribute to girls being less often identified with either autism or ADHD by their teachers, educational psychologists and even parents. Such work has reported and maintained a 'women (chiefly higher-functioning women) are missed' narrative that now runs through both autism and ADHD research, clinical practice and media coverage.[19, 21–29]

Recent sub-narratives to explain the missed-ness of women

The female autism phenotype

An influential narrative states that able females with autism are particularly under-recognised and have missed out on an autism diagnosis because their autistic behaviour and autistic traits are different from those of males with autism.[21] That is, there is a 'female autism phenotype' (FAP), a set of traits particular to women; *ergo*, there is also a male autism phenotype (MAP). In the FAP/MAP model, both men and women have underlying (biological) autism but their autism is expressed differently as they grow up due to social, developmental and environmental factors. Women and girls are missing from the statistics and miss out on diagnosis because the current diagnostic criteria and scales, such as Autism Diagnostic Observation Schedule (ADOS) and Autism Diagnostic Interview-Revised (ADI-r), were developed from earlier concepts of autism that were oriented towards MAP traits.[30] Men and children were preponderant in the samples underpinning diagnostic scales originally developed in the days of ICD-9/DSM-III.[31, 32]

If autism is delineated with reference to current diagnostic criteria and if the criteria of core autism are defined by MAP, autism is MAP. Therefore, FAP is not autism as we currently define it, but is something else, unless core autism is re-defined to include FAP, in which case autism becomes FAP + MAP. My point being that autism is currently defined by behaviour and we decide what that behaviour is, rather than there being an identifyable biological marker underpinning the word. This idea of FAP seems to be now playing out in UK clinical practice; clinicians in Jennie Hayes's studies declared that ADOS would not identify women, therefore ADOS results were over-ruled on the basis that they would not show FAP and therefore would not be valid for women.[33]

Scales that specifically recognise FAP are being developed. However, the pilot version of the Girls' Questionnaire for Autism Spectrum Conditions (the GS-ASC)[34] – the components of which include 'lack of gendered behaviour' and 'lack of compliance' would make any feminist cringe. It includes questions designed to identify autism in women: preferring boys' toys (footballs?) to girls' toys, lacking interest in fashion or not preferring to look 'feminine'. One might assume many girls like football, lack interest in fashion and reject 'looking feminine', without these being a sign of autism. Furthermore, the GS-ASC identifies adolescent girls' confusion about their sexuality as a sign of autism. Thus, the scale delivers a picture in which autism, oppressive gender norms and feminine stereotypes are unfortunately conflated. The interweaving of what counts as appropriate behaviour according to gender and what counts as autism is clearly challenging to disentangle.

Masking

A second persuasive narrative is that able women with autism have missed out on an autism diagnosis because they are able to effectively mask their autism. High-achieving women, it is thought, may be better at hiding their autism by imitating social interactions.[22, 35] 'Masking' is generally thought of as the way a person with autism (or any other social impairment) disguises their underlying 'true' self and passes as socially competent by using rote or learnt behaviours or acting in a socially acceptable way.

Masking is also known as camouflaging, acting or passing. Each term has slightly different connotations. The term 'passing' has been used by gay rights activists to describe passing as heterosexual;[36] for autism the analogy is 'passing' as neurotypical.[37] Passing is situationally employed to resist social oppression and can be considered as a social interaction strategy that is 'a performance in which one presents oneself as what one is not'.[38]

For autistic women, masking also means suppressing in public behaviours that are characteristic of autism, for example hand flapping or other repetitive movements. Our work on adults' experiences of repetitive movements, known as stimming, found that such movements were frequently suppressed in public, despite stimming's helpful function in the regulation of emotions,[39] a study I describe in more depth in a later chapter (Chapter 9). Masking can also involve the use of rote learning or mimicked behaviours to 'pass as normal' in initiating and maintaining social interactions. In a UK-based study exploring the broad phenomenon of masking, researchers reported women using masking and other compensation techniques to pretend to be like other women, as one woman said, to: 'put on my best normal'.[26] An ability to mask was mediated by how much energy people felt they could muster at any one time. In some cases, masking is a learned strategy that becomes almost automatic. In certain social spaces, women pass using the social and gendered signals that are expected in a given situation, such as acting sociably, being communicative or empathetic and being socially engaged at a party.[40]

The notion of masking behaviours poses problems for both feminist theory and for clinicians who are attempting to make diagnostic decisions. All women (and all men) adopt roles to fit into social interactions. All the world's a stage, and all women play characters in social spaces, be it mother, interviewee, work colleague, party guest or friend in the pub. The philosopher Judith Butler, in her feminist classic *Gender Trouble*,[41] argues that the notion of gender itself is a kind of improvised performance. How, then, is it possible to differentiate between autistic masking and a neurotypical (allistic) woman adopting a social role in her everyday life?

Masking is described in DSM-5 as a way for women and girls to disguise autism,[42] and is included as a component of the above-mentioned GQ-ASC scale. Masking (the ability to read social norms, be adept at fitting in and not have behaviours that are pervasive across settings) is thus almost the polar opposite of pre-1990 understanding of autism, in which *lack* of understanding of social norms and the omnipresence of autistic behaviours across settings were indicators. Today, as Hayes observed, fitting into social expectations (if at a cost and in a limited way), even if not unique to autism, is interpreted as a sign and used to diagnose autism in practice.[43] Butler argues that, if gender is performative, no identity exists behind the acts that supposedly 'express' gender and these acts constitute, rather than express, the illusion of the underlying stable gender identity.[42] Could the same be true for autism? Could interpretation as masking partially constitute the idea of a stable underlying autism? When a person is masking, passing for normal in diagnostic assessment, how can a clinician tell what their version of normal really is?

The idea of masking has caught the imagination of writers on social media, in women's magazines and mainstream newspapers and popular broadcasters.[44] Popular stories of missed or late-diagnosed autistic women are drawn from first-person accounts. Most are accounts of women diagnosed late in life who never realised they were autistic but to whom the diagnosis has been a revelation, with headlines such as '30 years trying to blend in', 'It all made sense when we found out we were autistic'[45] or 'The costs of camouflaging'.[46] Such sources serve to make the masking narrative culturally accessible and available.

Masking was examined in some depth in the British network television programme *Are You Autistic?*[40] The programme featured an experiment in which four women speed-dated young men. The women were adept at flirting, eye contact and initiating conversation. All the men they met felt comfortable and engaged. The men were amazed to learn their dates were autistic. This, we were told, was evidence of camouflaging or masking in the autistic women, who went on to describe how the effort to 'pass' was draining. Delineation between autistic and allistic masking was made on the basis of effort and recovery.

Misdiagnosis

A final narrative explaining the missing women contends that, partly because diagnostic criteria and diagnostic scales are geared toward picking up MAP and perhaps partly because autism is stereotyped as a 'male' condition, girls and women with FAP are either totally missed or misdiagnosed with other conditions,[19] often mental health conditions. Co-occurring conditions such as borderline/emotionally unstable personality disorder,[47] anxiety[48] and eating disorders[49] might conceal autism, or autistic women might be inappropriately labelled and thus never reach autism clinics.

'Mis'-diagnosis, however, assumes an autism diagnosis is a fixed constellation of behavioural traits that does not shift, with a 'correct' way of defining it, and that other psychiatric diagnoses have similarly fixed meanings, hence the mistaken classification. Historically, as different diagnoses go in and out of fashion and represent different constellations of symptoms, this model seems to be a red herring,[50] because previous diagnoses may have most accurately reflected the best understandings of women's difficulties at the time. Only recently has autism expanded to become an appropriate label for high-achieving women; once identified they are a new type of person as suggested by Hacking.[51] In this light, misdiagnosis is a misnomer. Perhaps the better question about any diagnosis is not 'is it correct?', for that alters with the flux of knowledge, but rather how *useful* is the diagnosis? (see Chapter 10).

Our study of autistic women and clinicians' perspectives

In 2019 and early 2020 I led a final qualitative study of women's accounts for *Exploring Diagnosis*. We gathered data from 31 first-person accounts that were previously published[52] and Jean Harrington, a sociologist, interviewed nine women (mostly by phone), with post-doc researcher Shelley Norman conducting follow-up interviews by e-mail due to Covid restrictions. I provided an inductive (theory-based) coding framework, which I applied together with Norman. With Harrington, I convened a discussion of masking at a clinician network meeting, in which approximately 30 clinicians from adult diagnostic services participated.

Most of the women in our interview sample were highly educated (often with post-graduate qualifications, including several with PhDs and one professor) and generally high achieving. Most had strongly autistic identities and most had actively sought an autism diagnosis. This was unsurprising, as our recruitment and sampling strategy called to those who wanted to write or speak about the transformative effect of a late diagnosis. All the women wrote or spoke articulately and most of those who gave their relationship status were in long-term relationships. This sample of women illustrates the difference between the very modern picture and the pre-1990s' version of autism, in which typically a diagnosis would be made for a male child with intellectual disability who might be non-verbal and have severe developmental delay.

We wanted to examine whether, and how, the women operationalised the autistic sub-narratives, to explore clinicians' perspectives and understand how gender norms and autism might intersect. More broadly, I wanted to find out what work an autism diagnosis did for the women, a slightly different focus to that of other groups.[21, 26, 53–55]

The preliminary findings showed many of the women felt a deep sense of alienation and 'otherness' before diagnosis, particularly in relation to gendered expectations. Together, they expressed a feeling that, from a young age, girls have more social expectations placed on them, and more value is placed on social abilities for women than men. A large proportion felt that, due merely to their sex, they were expected to conform to a submissive role and take on maternal, homemaking and caring duties. They also projected a feeling that their differences were highlighted and exacerbated by such gendered expectations. For some, their female sex left them feeling adrift from typical girls:

> *Little girls and bigger girls are supposed to chatter and giggle and gossip and share secrets and have best friends and so on … I didn't do that. My wiring (the neurological configuration of crucial parts of my brain) didn't let me (s7).*
>
> *I think it's harder for women, because we're expected to be more sociable, we're expected to fit that gender stereotype. So if you break out of that mould then*

you're seen as … I think, well, boys and men can get away with more without being called odd (J3).

The things other girls did and wanted to talk about held little interest for me … they wondered what was wrong with me … I am not into clothes or makeup or shopping, decorating, cooking all the things that seem so very important to them (S16).

One of the things that being a woman involves is the role of caregiver; the one who responds to needs, who nurtures … I am aware of the expectation … but I don't know what to do about it (S12).

In common with other studies,[53] many recounted being told they had something wrong with them: 'feeling like you're wrong, rather than feeling like something's wrong' (V6). The sense of 'otherness' was expressed as a feeling of being told one was not quite right, not fitting in, and so being subject to others' negative value judgements:

All my life there was a feeling of isolation … what's more I was always blamed for this. People would say 'if you could just enjoy the things other little girls enjoy, you would be much happier' (S23).

The women also said they did not think in the same way or use the same lens as those around them. This feeling of isolation and lack of being understood was counteracted by identification as autistic, mediated through the act of autism diagnosis. The label of autism not only gave them an explanation but also gave others a way to make their differences acceptable. The diagnosis embellished an 'illness narrative' (a term from medical sociology) through which to re-interpret their lives.[56-59] Diagnosis can be a turning point for framing one's own narrative – a form of biographical disruption.[60] Diagnosis allows a person to make sense of their experience and construct their story around it.

For many, though not all, diagnosis gave entry to a sense of place or community in which to understand themselves and their differences. As in a previous study, diagnosis was 'experienced by several participants as facilitating transition from being self-critical to self-compassionate, coupled with an increased sense of agency'.[53] The women experienced a change of identity that enabled greater acceptance and understanding of their self, positioning autism and its accompanying sub-narratives as an explanation for troubles rather than leading to any specific medical treatment or accessing of services. The healing power of diagnosis lay in its story telling and its ability to validate and legitimise difference:

[Diagnosis] claimed my right to actually be here, it legitimised it, I suppose or it created a space that I was entirely entitled to (J8).

It has changed just about everything. It has made it easier for me to forgive myself for the things I find difficult and mistakes I have made, things that have gone wrong … it is very helpful in allowing me to frame and contextualise some of my personality traits, actions and experiences (J11).

Narrative reconstruction involved resistance to normalising ideology. The autism diagnosis allowed the women to act in ways that might otherwise be unacceptable. It allowed them not to conform:

> It's just liberating and it really takes the pressure off ... I can withdraw from this situation because it's too much for me and it gives me permission really. Because without that sort of diagnosis, people just expect me to be one way (V3).

For these high-achieving women, an autism diagnosis had the effect of substituting a neuro-explanation for what might previously have been seen as their personal responsibility or failing. In this sense, diagnosis exculpated them from others' judgement of not living up to social norms:

> It's made me feel a lot better about myself, definitely ... yes, you have these difficulties for this reason, you are not just some kind of oddball, your autistic brain is different ... it explains it, it validates it almost ... it's an actual condition that I have no control over really, I can't change how I am (J7).

Diagnosis helped exempt the women from the expectations of traditional female roles. The liminal nature of these women's previous experience of being outsiders was replaced by a sense of relief, and sometimes a confirmed place in the thriving autistic community.

The missing-ness of women with autism was another topic, which participants largely related to their experience of going undetected or undiagnosed for a long time. Experiences were interpreted in the light of FAP and several women recounted that they were misdiagnosed with mental health conditions, which they found stigmatising, before settling on what they regarded as the useful, and correct, autism diagnosis.

There were numerous accounts of masking, styled as acting a role to fit in and disguise differences that the women felt were innate. They also used words such as passing, acting, adopting personae or mimicking. UK participants more often used the notion of 'masking' to describe attempts to fit in, remain undetected as autistic or act in gendered social spaces. This might have been because masking is named and identified in many culturally accessible narratives in the UK (such as the *Are You Autistic?* flirting experiment).

> I don't know how good boys are at masking but I just feel that my camouflaging, my masking, is brilliant, because I can go into a place and nobody will know I'm autistic (J4).
>
> For years, I tried desperately to conform and fit in and be one of the gang (S1).
>
> If you're like me and you're intelligent enough to memorise what other people do and try and mask, blend in ... you just do it, you're just pretending to be like the other people (J5).

The women described carefully studying others to develop their masks and how it took a large amount of energy to put on and wear them, and that they needed time to recover afterwards. Diagnosis absolved them from having to wear a mask:

> With the diagnosis it's that I'm free of that now because whatever people say is people judge me, it doesn't matter any more because officially I don't have to be like they expect me to be ... it was about a need to be my true self (J3).

The women provided insights that I was not expecting. Regarding parenting, there was a strong sense of the benefits of being a neurodivergent parent with a neurodivergent child; they felt able to relate to their children's perceptions of the world. Some said their autistic identities led them to reduce the expectations for their children to be something they were not, to have fewer expectations of what the child 'should' be like, particularly with respect to gendered norms and milestones. This might allow their children to grow up in a more positive environment than they themselves had experienced.

Interestingly, despite their academic achievements, and being outwardly perceived as successful, the women often recounted carrying a sense of failure. This may have been due to internalising, in their youth, the messages of not fitting in and having something wrong with them. They saw success as having a personal expense, in terms of the energy it took to continually keep wearing 'the mask' and be accepted. Some women felt that their abilities and strengths in the academic realm seeded expectations to be socially successful. They felt that others opined they were capable, so must simply not be trying, socially.

Underscoring earlier points about the situated nature of a need for diagnosis, some of the women described how profound life changes, such as divorce or losing a job, had led to the need for diagnosis becoming more pressing, as they were less supported. Looking at dementia, Baptiste Brossard and Normand Carpentier showed how perturbations in social networks can lead to diagnosis, as well as flow from it.[61] Bereavement, moving house or losing one's job may all prompt the interpretation of troubles (they define 'troubles' as social support interacting with impairment) in a diagnostic frame, prompting diagnosis, often so as to access additional support. This was true also for several of the parents in one of my first studies, who described a 'tipping point' created by circumstances such as school transition, that led them to pursue an autism diagnosis for their child.[62] Autism needed to be named only in relation to expectation, support received and social difficulties.

To recap, in common with the FAP study,[21] many women felt they did not 'fit in' to the profile of a typical girl or traditional ideas about femininity, and used their autism diagnosis as an explanation for their differences. Autism diagnosis had a healing role and provided an explanation for a lifetime of difference, as seen elsewhere,[26, 53] and in other conditions,[56, 61] enabled them to disrupt or reposition their biography and gave a sense of community and belonging. All three sub-narratives – missing, masking and misdiagnosis – were operationalised to storify and interpret experiences.

Clinicians' perspectives

Conversations with clinicians in adult assessment services about masking and aut-istic identity led to questions about how the clinicians identified 'autistic' masking (as opposed to everyday gendered and social roles). The clinicians' responses elaborated on the question:

> *Is it the quality of the masking? … Or is it the degree of effort needed and the exhaustion? … and how are each of these features different to those in neurotypicals? So do I diagnose a person as ASD [autism spectrum disorder] if they say they have to have 30 minutes to themselves to calm down when they get home or should it be 2 hours? Or is time irrelevant and the reasons that matter – what reasons are we looking for? With all of this so varied depending on intelligence, self awareness and support levels through life is for me a fascin-ating question.*

(Psychiatrist, 2019)

At a meeting of UK autism adult assessment services in 2019, clinicians described how they could differentiate autistic masking from gendered and social role play, because masking behaviours were learnt or scripted. Clinicians also cited the increased recovery time for masking. Autistic masking might also involve elab-orate efforts, for example laborious, perhaps months-long, planning for an event. Clinicians reported using their judgement and expertise to differentiate between allistic masking and autistic masking. Allistic people, they said, navigated social interaction more intuitively, whereas a higher-functioning autistic woman might adopt a logical approach.

However, some clinicians talked of their exasperation, those 'heart sink moments' when women with strong autistic identities, who clearly were not aut-istic in the clinicians' eyes, claimed their autism could not be identified because 'Yes, I'm socially skilled but I'm masking'. Masking had caused a re-thinking of what signifies autism. In borderline cases, those 'on the verge', in the sub-clinical, threshold region, clinicians were struggling to identify who 'really' had autism: the problem was 'how to turn a smudged line into a real one', as one psychiatrist put it. The clinicians said that an alternative diagnosis might be more appropriate, as other mental health conditions also involve masking. I have myself witnessed my mother increasingly use rote and scripted social conversation to mask her progressing dementia. As she struggles to think of things to say, she falls back on repeating known patterns of conversation that have served her well throughout her life. The clinicians pointed out that neurotypical people also 'act roles through [a] desire to save face' and/or fit in. Women's experience of 'other-ness', they pointed out, could be due to myriad causes, not only autism; people who had experienced depression, or trauma, also felt 'different'. The issue was where the feeling stemmed from; getting the correct formulation was tricky.

Nevertheless, in diagnostic spaces, both clinicians and clients invoked masking as evidence of autism in women.[33] Diagnostic services require autism to be a recognisable entity that is pervasive across settings. If autism is pervasive, a person cannot have autism in one situation and not in another. Masking allowed autistic women to behave in a non-autistic way in some contexts but not in others. For high-achieving women at a fuzzy boundary, the question clinicians had to answer (due to institutional demands) was if woman X had autism or not. It takes work to create and maintain a real, defendable boundary between who has autism and who does not; clinicians occasionally used the masking narrative to help protect it. Autism sub-narratives were operationalised in clinical practice to help steer and account for decisions, yet simultaneously questioned outside the diagnostic space.

The clinicians discussed how autism in adults has become a more positive identity, making it a preferable diagnosis to, for example, personality disorder. Autism, they pointed out, is more socially acceptable nowadays than it was in 1990, at least in the UK, which is partly due to de-stigmatisation (see Chapter 4), including the very public testimony of the healing power of autism diagnosis in the written testimonies we reviewed.[52] The act of de-stigmatising the category meant other women would be more likely to adopt the label in future. Looping, again.

The clinicians felt deeply uncomfortable about having to 'police identities', questioning whether 'we really have the right to do this?' Some of the clients coming to adult assessment services were convinced of their autism and had strong autistic identities. Others had equally strong non-autistic identities. Clinicians recounted instances in which they saw clients who strongly self-identified as autistic but were not diagnosed, which felt tantamount to denying the person their identity. Some clinicians had been accused of epistemic violence by *not* giving a diagnosis and, in some cases, clients had threatened to kill themselves. 'We are challenging people's sense of self', said one clinician. This was really a social issue, not a medical one, and not part of their professional role, they felt.

The *Exploring Diagnosis* interviews included a woman who self-identified as autistic who, when a diagnosis was not granted, simply discounted her clinical assessors as wrong. The assessors did not understand autism or masking, she concluded. A second woman with a strong autistic identity simply shopped around until she found a clinician in private practice who was prepared to confirm the diagnosis that she wanted. In some cases, there also seemed to be a level of performance during assessment: performing autism, almost. This is perhaps not surprising if they were practised actors; they were performing autism to get the diagnosis they desired:

> *You have to go in to the [clinic] and make a sales pitch and it's got to be convincing or they're not going to let you do it (J5).*

Clinicians described clients who, before assessment, engaged with forums and academic literature to find out what autism is. They felt clients with a strong identity did, to some extent, 'perform autism' (or not) to achieve the diagnostic outcome they wanted. We saw similar evidence of performing to achieve the desired outcome in our 2012 study, in which I interviewed some parents who were resisting a diagnosis for their child, using 'engineering' and 'spin' to avoid a diagnosis:

> *I've coached her to be normal. She appears so much better than she is. I still believe I could play it any way I wanted to. You could play it so the opposite way and I absolutely would've done if we hadn't had enough money ... If you actually don't want your child to be diagnosed as autistic ... it's very difficult to answer them completely honestly. I think this is semi-subconscious, I didn't sit there thinking, 'I'm going to fake this' (mother of undiagnosed child).*

Stories, especially diagnostic narratives, are not neutral descriptions but themselves shape the diagnostic categories and help form our interpretations of our own experience. In the last chapter, I referred to the rise of culturally accessible narratives, anorexia in Japan (mentioned in the previous chapter) being an example, of a prevailing diagnostic narrative leading girls to newly express their distress through eating patterns, rather than through other behaviours.[63] There are power dynamics at play in the relative influence of these stories, as David Harper points out:

> *In mental health services there are a number of stakeholders' voices which need to be attended to: professionals of various disciplines; users of services; users' relatives; care staff; neighbours and so on. A social constructionist position would acknowledge that there are a variety of stories to be told but, when linked to a political analysis we must also acknowledge that some stories (e.g. those of professionals) are more powerful than others (e.g. those of service users). The decision about how to deal with these stories is a political one.[64]*

Masking, missing-ness and misdiagnosis are discussed 'in-group' in texts such as those we drew on but also in on-line autism chat rooms, where the stories are iterated, repeated, recognised and reified.[65] These virtual meeting spaces and public accounts not only help members and readers to locate and make meaning of their own experience but also co-constitute experience with others, providing the tools to experience it differently. The shared stories provide a point of connection and belonging.[65, 66] Locating oneself as autistic, rewriting biography in the light of diagnosis, is so important for some that it seems to seed a form of autistic fundamentalism, an unwavering attachment to the belief in autism, a strong emphasis on in-group and out-group distinctions, accompanied by quasi-religious enlightenment: 'when I got my diagnosis it all made sense'.[45] Contrary views can be experienced as an attack on selfhood or community.[67] The situation is reminiscent of the wider debates around censorship and denial of personhood that have risen in the trans-exclusionary radical feminist debates and other forms of identity politics. Such polarisation between who is 'in' and who is 'out' has been critiqued as divisive and unhelpful.[68]

Gender and autism

For women, there seems to be an uneasy intersection between gender and autism. Issues of gender conformity and autism, lack of social conformity and sexuality seem conflated. An embodiment model, in which gender is performed, must incorporate hypotheses about initial biological vulnerabilities to autism – which may be differentially distributed in relation to biological sex – and their interactions with gender relations.[69] Social theorists outline that both hegemonic masculinity and hegemonic femininity are implicated in, and intersect with, other systems of inequality, such as disability.[70] There are clearly multi-faceted bio-logical, psychological, social and bio-political interactions between autism and gender.[69]

Some women, as evidenced by our study, felt pressured to conform to gen-dered social norms. Masking was one way to conform to such expectations. A diagnosis of autism provides explanation, exculpation and exemption from 'deviant' gendered behaviour, as some of their testimonies witnessed. Obtaining an autism diagnosis gave relief, as they were thus excused from moral obligations to perform a typical 'womanly' or feminine role: being sociable, making small talk, caring, putting others' needs first, and so on.

Setting a 'new normal'

In the context of their lived experience of the (normative) social rules, the idea of a person's 'normal' was re-set by diagnosis, to a new autistic normal that was less demanding, less restrictive and more tolerant of unusual social behaviour. The re-setting to a 'new normal' has been seen in studies of disclosure of diagnosis.[71] Disclosure may lead to fewer negative evaluations of a child displaying autistic behaviour but simultaneously lower people's expectations.[71-73]

The notion of a 'new normal' for expected behaviour was a phrase used in the UK and other countries as populations were locked down in response to the Covid-19 pandemic; new standards of behaviour were supported by shifts in infrastructure and the emergence of rules about social distancing, staying at home, on-line meetings, and so on, mostly policed by the community and through self-surveillance. This has been a shift in population-wide norms and expectations of behaviour required in response to risk. In contrast, norms that are shifted by the autistic frame are individualised norms of social conduct and the autistic frame creates a new normal in which deviant behaviour is more, not less, tolerated. Anecdotally we have heard that some people with autistic traits relish the solitude and on-line communication necessitated by lockdown. Perhaps the shift in population norms has bought one form of autistic cognitive style nearer the centre. What is considered population-normal can be fluid too.

The political consequence of diagnostic creep (Figure 3.1) into previously sub-clinical populations, such as high-achieving women and men, remains that increased diagnosis inadvertently contributes to a 'shrinking normal' for the allistic (non-autistic) group.[74] If 'healthy' is defined by its opposition to pathological or diagnosable,[75] the boundary of what is healthy/normal shrinks as medicalisation expands what can be diagnosed. By adopting exemption via diagnosis, expanding definitions of illness reconfigure – shrink – the underlying category of 'normality'.[76] If a woman's 'deviance' or lack of compliance is understood through exemption via autism diagnosis, conformist behaviour strengthens its grasp on allistic people; non-traditionally feminine behaviour becomes a sign of autism, for example, rather than an alternative acceptable form of normal behaviour for women. Diagnostic exemption gives norms the oxygen to tighten their grip on the shrinking normal. Some women seek a new identity to explain their personal experiences and difficulties. But an autism diagnosis is only one framework, one lens through which a coherent narrative,[58] and sense of relief, can be found by setting a 'new' normal.[78] Diagnosis is not the only way to storify a biography as I will discuss in the next chapter.

From the standpoints of diversity or feminism, it might be preferable to widen the ways all women (indeed, all people) are allowed or expected to behave. 'Feminine' traits are not fixed but rather are heavily constructed by social norms and power relations.[78] A more progressive social model would widen what constitutes 'deviant' femaleness; acceptable ways to be a girl should include being asocial, struggling with small talk, not feeling a nurturing instinct, not adopting caring roles and finding make-up and shopping uninspiring, with no need for a diagnosis of disorder. The feminist theorist, Mimi Schippers, writes of hegemonic femininity, meaning traits such as compliance, nurturing and empathy. These, she explains, have become associated with female sex, which legitimises men's dominance over women when paired with characteristics that supposedly differentiate men and women – such hegemonic masculine traits as assertiveness, physical strength and self-promotion. The women in our study operated a biological understanding to claim the new autistic normal (in Schippers's terms, creating a pariah femininity). In short, many traits various women in our study described as autistic were non-hegemonically feminine.[70]

Ideally, we would seek to overturn this system by replacing judgement with acceptance. But diagnosis is needed when acceptance is lacking. Diagnosis allows people to accept pariah femininity because it effectively reduces one's complex behaviours to facets of one's brain. By invoking diagnostic exceptionalism, the range of behaviour considered 'normal' in non-diagnosed women is maintained. Diagnosis therefore reinforces the rules for the majority and shores up gendered norms and values. The re-working of individual women's difficulties in 'fitting in' to a diagnosable disorder helps them adjust to the conditions that caused their problems but it does not set the rest of the population free.

The testimony of the women in our study also raised the question of whether men are equally likely to mask to fit in to traditional masculine roles. Our study did not include men, so this question is outside my scope. Anecdotally, a trans male-to-female autistic person reported that their asocial qualities were tolerated better as a man than as a woman. Possibly, if asocial behaviours are less stigmatised in men, men either feel less inclined to mask or try to fit in in different ways to

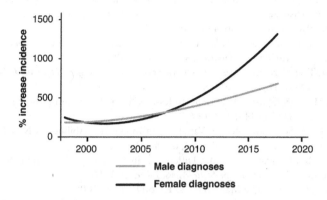

Figure 5.1 Percentage increase in incidence of autism diagnosis from 1998 to 2018 by gender.

women. The study of masking, how it and what else counts as autism, what counts as feminine and masculine and how this interacts with culture and masking is a promising area for future research.

Masking, misdiagnosis and the missed-ness of women are now established, recognised problems in today's autism landscape but only since the later twentieth century. Sub-narratives about women with autism not only passively reflect the facts but also have partially constituted the story. They have contributed to new understandings of autism and how it takes a different form in women. It seems stories of missing, masking and misdiagnosis are having an impact. Our analysis of general practitioner (GP) data showed a striking increase in the diagnosis of women, compared to men, since the early 2000s (Figure 5.1). (Note that the baseline of 1998 is held at the same level for women and men but far more men were diagnosed each year; the graph illustrates the *pace* of increase of diagnosis of women compared to men.)

I think it is inaccurate to think that women were 'missed' in the 1990s, because the boundaries of autism have moved. The women the clinicians described as 'on the verge' would not have been diagnosed then, because concepts of autism were narrower; autism meant something different. Autism has only recently become a condition that encompasses fluent, financially independent, successful women in long-term relationships. Women who may have been considered 'on the verge' in 2010 now qualify for diagnosis.

References

1. Fombonne, E. Epidemiology of Pervasive Developmental Disorders. *Pediatr. Res.* **65**, 591–598 (2009).
2. Wing, L. Sex Ratios in Early Childhood Autism and Related Conditions. *Psychiatry Res.* **5**, 129–137 (1981).

3. Loomes, R., Hull, L. & Mandy, W. P. L. What is the Male-to-Female Ratio in Autism Spectrum Disorder? A Systematic Review and Meta-Analysis. *J. Am. Acad. Child Adolesc. Psychiatry* **56**, 466–474 (2017).

4. Volkmar, F. R., Szatmari, P. & Sparrow, S. S. Sex Differences in Pervasive Developmental Disorders. *J. Autism Dev. Disord.* **23**, 579–591 (1993).

5. Brugha, T. *et al. Autism Spectrum Disorders in Adults Living in Households Throughout England.* (NHS Digital, 2009).

6. Marco, E. J. & Skuse, D. H. Autism-lessons from the X Chromosome. *Soc. Cogn. Affect. Neurosci.* **1**, 183–193 (2006).

7. Feingold, A. Sex Differences in Variability in Intellectual Abilities: A New Look at an Old Controversy. *Rev. Educ. Res.* **62**, 61–84 (1992).

8. Baye, A. & Monseur, C. Gender Differences in Variability and Extreme Scores in an International Context. *Large-Scale Assess. Educ.* **4** (2016).

9. Kraemer, S. The Fragile Male. *BMJ* **321**, 1609–1612 (2000).

10. Robinson, E. B., Lichtenstein, P., Anckarsater, H., Happe, F. & Ronald, A. Examining and Interpreting the Female Protective Effect Against Autistic Behavior. *Proc. Natl Acad. Sci.* **110**, 5258–5262 (2013).

11. Carazo, P., Green, J., Sepil, I., Pizzari, T. & Wigby, S. Inbreeding Removes Sex Differences in Lifespan in a Population of *Drosophila melanogaster. Biol. Lett.* **12**, 20160337 (2016).

12. Muenchhoff, M. & Goulder, P. J. R. Sex Differences in Pediatric Infectious Diseases. *J. Infect. Dis.* **209**, S120–S126 (2014).

13. Baron-Cohen, S. The Extreme Male Brain Theory of Autism. *Trends Cogn. Sci.* **6**, 248–254 (2002).

14. Knickmeyer, R., Baron-Cohen, S., Raggatt, P., Taylor, K. & Hackett, G. Fetal Testosterone and Empathy. *Horm. Behav.* **49**, 282–292 (2006).

15. Kaminsky, Z., Wang, S.-C. & Petronis, A. Complex Disease, Gender and Epigenetics. *Ann. Med.* **38**, 530–544 (2006).

16. Kreiser, N. L. & White, S. W. ASD in Females: Are We Overstating the Gender Difference in Diagnosis? *Clin. Child Fam. Psychol. Rev.* **17**, 67–84 (2014). doi:10.1007/s10567-013-0148-9.

17. Biederman, J. *et al.* Absence of Gender Effects on Attention Deficit Hyperactivity Disorder: Findings in Nonreferred Subjects. *Am. J. Psychiatry* **162**, 1083–1089 (2005).

18. Adams, C. Girls and ADHD: Are You Missing the Signs? *Instructor* **116**, 31–35 (2007).

19. Gould, J. & Ashton-Smith, J. Missed Diagnosis or Misdiagnosis? Girls and Women on the Autism Spectrum. www.ingentaconnect.com/content/bild/gap/2011/00000012/00000001/art00005 (2011).

20. Russell, G., Steer, C. & Golding, J. Social and Demographic Factors that Influence the Diagnosis of Autistic Spectrum Disorders. *Soc. Psychiatry Psychiatr. Epidemiol.* **46**, 1283–1293 (2011).

21. Bargiela, S., Steward, R. & Mandy, W. The Experiences of Late-diagnosed Women with Autism Spectrum Conditions: An Investigation of the Female Autism Phenotype. *J. Autism Dev. Disord.* **46**, 3281–3294 (2016).

22. Brugha, T. S. *et al.* Epidemiology of Autism in Adults Across Age Groups and Ability Levels. *Br. J. Psychiatry* **209**, 498–503 (2016).

23. Coles, E. K., Slavec, J., Bernstein, M. & Baroni, E. Exploring the Gender Gap in Referrals for Children with ADHD and Other Disruptive Behavior Disorders. *J. Atten. Disord.* **16**, 101–108 (2012).

24. Groenewald, C., Emond, A. & Sayal, K. Recognition and Referral of Girls with Attention Deficit Hyperactivity Disorder: Case Vignette Study. *Child Care Health Dev.* **35**, 767–772 (2009).

25. Holtmann, M., Bölte, S. & Poustka, F. Autism Spectrum Disorders: Sex Differences in Autistic Behaviour Domains and Coexisting Psychopathology. *Dev. Med. Child Neurol.* **49**, 361–366 (2007).

26. Hull, L. *et al.* 'Putting on My Best Normal': Social Camouflaging in Adults with Autism Spectrum Conditions. *J. Autism Dev. Disord.* **47**, 2519–2534 (2017).

27. Rucklidge, J. J. Gender Differences in Attention-deficit/Hyperactivity Disorder. *Psychiatr. Clin. North Am.* **33**, 357–373 (2010).

28. Sciutto, M. J., Nolfi, C. J. & Bluhm, C. Effects of Child Gender and Symptom Type on Referrals for ADHD by Elementary School Teachers. *J. Emot. Behav. Disord.* **12**, 247–253 (2004).

29. Sturm, H., Fernell, E. & Gillberg, C. Autism Spectrum Disorders in Children with Normal Intellectual Levels: Associated Impairments and Subgroups. *Dev. Med. Child Neurol.* **46**, 444–447 (2004).

30. Haney, J. L. Autism, Females, and the DSM-5: Gender Bias in Autism Diagnosis. *Soc. Work Ment. Health* **14**, 396–407 (2016).

31. Lord, C., Rutter, M. & Le Couteur, A. Autism Diagnostic Interview-Revised: A Revised Version of a Diagnostic Interview for Caregivers of Individuals with Possible Pervasive Developmental Disorders. *J. Autism Dev. Disord.* **24**, 659–685 (1994).

32. Lord, C., Risi, S. & Lambrecht, L. The Autism Diagnostic Observation Schedule-Generic; A Standard Measure of Social and Communication Deficits Associated with the Spectrum of Autism. *J Autism Dev Disord* **30**, 205–233 (2000).

33. Hayes, J., McCabe, R., Ford, T. & Russell, G. Drawing a Line in the Sand: Affect and Testimony in Autism Assessment Teams in the UK. *Sociol. Health Illn.* **42**, 825–843 (2020).

34. GQ-ASC: Girls' Questionnaire for Autism Spectrum Conditions. *Minds & Hearts.* https://mindsandhearts.net/gq-asc-girls-questionnaire-for-autism-spectrum-conditions/.

35. Willey, L. H. *Pretending to be Normal: Living with Asperger's Syndrome* (Jessica Kingsley Publishers, 1999).

36. Kalei Kanuha, V. The Social Process of Passing to Manage Stigma: Acts of Internalized Oppression of Acts of Resistance. *J. Sociol. Soc. Welf.* **26**, 27 (1999).

37. Scuro, J. *Addressing Ableism: Philosophical Questions via Disability Studies* (Lexington Books, 2017).

38. Ginsberg, E. K. & Pease, D. E. *Passing and the Fictions of Identity* (Duke University Press, 1996).

39. Kapp, S. K. *et al.* 'People Should be Allowed to Do What They Like': Autistic Adults' Views and Experiences of Stimming. *Autism* **23**, 1782–1792 (2019). doi:10.1177/1362361319829628.

40. Channel 4. Are You Autistic? www.channel4.com/press/news/are-you-autistic (2018).

41. Butler, J. *Gender Trouble* (Routledge, 2006).

42. American Psychiatric Association & DSM-5 Task Force. *Diagnostic and Statistical Manual of Mental Disorders: DSM-5* (American Psychiatric Association, 2013).

43. Hayes, J. Drawing a Line in the Sand: Autism Diagnosis as Social Process. PhD thesis. https://ore.exeter.ac.uk/repository/bitstream/handle/10871/120580/HayesJ.pdf?sequence=1&isAllowed=y (2020).

44. Ploszajski, A. Women 'Better than Men at Disguising Autism Symptoms'. *The Guardian* (13 September 2019).

45. BBC. It All Made Sense When We Found Out We Were Autistic. www.bbc.co.uk/news/resources/idt-sh/women_late_diagnosis_autism (2019).

46. Russo, F. Spectrum. The Costs of Camouflaging Autism. www.spectrumnews.org/features/deep-dive/costs-camouflaging-autism/ (2018).

47. Rydén, G., Rydén, E. & Hetta, J. Borderline Personality Disorder and Autism Spectrum Disorder in Females: A Cross-sectional Study. *Clin. Neuropsychiatry J. Treat. Eval.* **5**, 22–30 (2008).

48. Kerns, C. M. & Kendall, P. C. The Presentation and Classification of Anxiety in Autism Spectrum Disorder. *Clin. Psychol. Sci. Pract.* **19**, 323–347 (2012).

49. Nilsson, E. W., Gillberg, C., Gillberg, I. C. & Råstam, M. Ten-year Follow-up of Adolescent-onset Anorexia Nervosa: Personality Disorders. *J. Am. Acad. Child Adolesc. Psychiatry* **38**, 1389–1395 (1999).

50. Russell, G. & Ford, T. The Costs and Benefits of Diagnosis of ADHD: Commentary on Holden et al. *Child Adolesc. Psychiatry Ment. Health* **8**, 7 (2014).

51. Hacking, I. Making Up People. *London Review of Books* **28**, 23–26 (2006).

52. Miller, J. K. *Women From Another Planet?: Our Lives in the Universe of Autism* (AuthorHouse, 2003).

53. Leedham, A., Thompson, A. R., Smith, R. & Freeth, M. 'I was Exhausted Trying to Figure it Out': The Experiences of Females Receiving an Autism Diagnosis in Middle to Late Adulthood. *Autism* **24**, 135–146 (2020).

54. Livingston, L. A., Shah, P. & Happé, F. Compensatory Strategies Below the Behavioural Surface in Autism: A Qualitative Study. *Lancet Psychiatry* **6**, 766–777 (2019).

55. Tint, A. & Weiss, J. A. A Qualitative Study of the Service Experiences of Women with Autism Spectrum Disorder. *Autism* **22**, 928–937 (2018).

56. Huibers, M. J. H. & Wessely, S. The Act of Diagnosis: Pros and Cons of Labelling Chronic Fatigue Syndrome. *Psychol. Med.* **36**, 895–900 (2006).

57. Riessman, C. K. Strategic Uses of Narrative in the Presentation of Self and Illness: A Research Note. *Soc. Sci. Med. 1982* **30**, 1195–1200 (1990).

58. Smith, B. & Sparkes, A. C. Changing Bodies, Changing Narratives and the Consequences of Tellability: A Case Study of Becoming Disabled Through Sport. *Sociol. Health Illn.* **30**, 217–236 (2008).

59. Frank, A. W. Just Listening: Narrative and Deep Illness. *Fam. Syst. Health* **16**, 197–212 (1998).

60. Bury, M. Chronic Illness as Biographical Disruption. *Sociol. Health Illn.* **4**, 167–182 (1982).

61. Brossard, B. & Carpentier, N. To What Extent Does Diagnosis Matter? Dementia Diagnosis, Trouble Interpretation and Caregiving Network Dynamics. *Sociol. Health Illn.* **39**, 566–580 (2017).

62. Russell, G. & Norwich, B. Dilemmas, Diagnosis and De-stigmatization: Parental Perspectives on the Diagnosis of Autism Spectrum Disorders. *Clin. Child Psychol. Psychiatry* **17**, 229–245 (2012).

63. Watters, E. *Crazy Like Us: The Globalization of the American Psyche* (Free Press, 2010).

64. Harper, D. J. Discourse Analysis and 'Mental Health'. *J Ment. Health* **4**, 347–358 (1995).

65. Davidson, J. Autistic Culture Online: Virtual Communication and Cultural Expression on the Spectrum. *Soc. Cult. Geogr.* **9**, 791–806 (2008).

66. Davidson, J. & Henderson, V. L. 'Travel in Parallel with us for a While': Sensory Geographies of Autism. *Can. Geogr. Géographe Can.* **54**, 462–475 (2010).

67. Guest, E. Autism from Different Points of View: Two Sides of the Same Coin. *Disabil. Soc.* **0**, 1–7 (2019).

68. Russell, G. Critiques of the Neurodiversity Movement. In *Autistic Community and the Neurodiversity Movement: Stories from the Frontline* (ed. Kapp, S. K.) 287–303 (Springer, 2020). doi:10.1007/978-981-13-8437-0_21.

69. Cheslack-Postava, K. & Jordan-Young, R. M. Autism Spectrum Disorders: Toward a Gendered Embodiment Model. *Soc. Sci. Med. 1982* **74**, 1667–1674 (2012).

70. Schippers, M. Recovering the Feminine Other: Masculinity, Femininity, and Gender Hegemony. *Theory Soc.* **36**, 85–102 (2007).

71. Sasson, N. J. & Morrison, K. E. First Impressions of Adults with Autism Improve with Diagnostic Disclosure and Increased Autism Knowledge of Peers. *Autism* **23**, 50–59 (2019).

72. Chambres, P., Auxiette, C., Vansingle, C. & Gil, S. Adult Attitudes Toward Behaviors of a Six-year-old Boy with Autism. *J. Autism Dev. Disord.* **38**, 1320–1327 (2008).

73. White, R. *et al.* Is Disclosing an Autism Spectrum Disorder in School Associated with Reduced Stigmatization? *Autism* **24**, 744–754 (2020) doi:10.1177/1362361319887625.

74. Frances, A. *Saving Normal: An Insider's Revolt Against Out-of-Control Psychiatric Diagnosis, DSM-5, Big Pharma, and the Medicalization of Ordinary Life* (HarperCollins, 2014).

75. Jutel, A. & Nettleton, S. Towards a Sociology of Diagnosis: Reflections and Opportunities. *Soc. Sci. Med. 1982* **73**, 793–800 (2011).

76. Sweet, P. L. & Decoteau, C. L. Contesting Normal: The DSM-5 and Psychiatric Subjectivation. *BioSocieties* **13**, 103–122 (2018).

77. Mallett, R. & Runswick Cole, K. How Impairment Labels Function. In *Theorising Normalcy and the Mundane: Precarious Positions* (eds Mallett, R, Ogden, C. A., & Slater, J.) (University of Chester Press, 2016).

78. Kalof, L. Dilemmas of Femininity: Gender and the Social Construction of Sexual Imagery. *Sociol. Q.* **34**, 639–651 (1993).

6 Beyond the living

What do Hans Christian Andersen, Steve Jobs and Marie Curie have in common? They have all been retrospectively diagnosed with autism. Anyone with a passing interest in autism might have noticed the media flurry accompanying 'diagnoses' of dead historical figures, celebrities or fictional characters. This is psychopathography, the process of retrofitting a mental disorder after someone has died.[1]

One reason there are so many excellent candidates for retrospective diagnosis of autism is its current heterogeneity. Autistic traits are hugely varied; it has become a loose and flexible category that, combined with hazy and elastic interpretations of the historical source evidence (diaries, artefacts, anecdotal accounts, biographies, and even pottery) makes extra-clinical diagnosis easy to apply.

The retrospective diagnosis of autism illustrates a general enthusiasm for autism, a diagnostic *zeitgeist*. Together with Katherine Foxhall,[2] we have argued that retrospective diagnosis tells us little about the person diagnosed and more about the era the diagnosers live in, and the dominance of diagnostic frameworks.[1]

The godfather of retrospective autism diagnosis is Michael Fitzgerald, a professor of child and adolescent psychiatry, who has made numerous retrospective diagnoses of autism in his books. He claims Lewis Carroll, Éamon de Valera, Sir Keith Joseph, Ramanujan, WB Yeats, Hans Christian Andersen, George Orwell and even Adolf Hiltler as autistic.[3, 4] Other recent examples are Field Marshall Montgomery (1887–1976), diagnosed by the historian Antony Beevor,[5] and the walker and writer Alfred Wainwright (1907–1991), diagnosed in the biography by the journalist Richard Else.[6]

Fitzgerald offers a detailed diagnosis with reference to the philosopher Ludwig Wittgenstein, who was originally described as on the spectrum by Gillberg.[6] Fitzgerald matches descriptions of Wittgenstein's teaching techniques and reports of his cold personality with diagnostic criteria, describing philosophy as Wittgenstein's special interest, pursued to the exclusion of other activities.[7] According to Fitzgerald, Wittgenstein 'certainly did have a desire to interact with others in relation to his special interest, philosophy' but at the same time 'did not need philosophical co-workers' ([7] p. 62). This somewhat conflicting account illustrates the difficulty in pinning down what signifies autism and the difficulty in diagnosis stemming from an open re-interpretation of a second-hand account.

But this does not mean the diagnosis is incorrect in today's terms. We can never know if Wittgenstein would have qualified for an autism diagnosis today, were he alive, or indeed whether he would have sought one.

Chris Timms criticises the retrospective autism diagnosis as applied to Field Marshall Montgomery, although he stops short of stating there was no autism as we know it in Monty's lifetime.[8] Timms suggests Montgomery's lack of empathy was typical of a military leader of his time and argues the use of evidence to diagnose Montgomery as autistic is highly selective and ignores conflicting data. Montgomery's diagnostic story gives descriptions of events in his life a meaningful causal framework; in particular, the autism diagnosis provides a narrative frame to explain and classify Monty's aberrant social communication and work-focused behaviour.

Popular texts have diagnosed many other historical figures with autism. The website *History's 30 Most Inspiring People on the Autism Spectrum* claims both celebrities and historical figures, offering a short paragraph of evidence for each case to support the diagnosis of, among others, Charles Darwin, Stanley Kubrick, Michelangelo, Mozart, Sir Isaac Newton and the film director Tim Burton (based on an assessment by his ex-wife, Helena Bonham Carter). The wide range of signs and indicators cited as evidence by the diagnosers gives autism a catch-all tinge, allowing the use of autism as a generic explanation for deviance from a wide range of norms.

Retrospective diagnosis of autism is also used to provide encouragement and create inspirational role models for autistic children. The best-selling children's book *Different Like Me: My Book of Autism Heroes* lists Einstein, Warhol, Kandinsky, Turing, Tesla and Immanuel Kant as on the spectrum.[9] By describing the amazing achievements of the historical figures deemed autistic, the book's aim is to inspire and motivate children told they have autism.

Steve Jobs, the founder of Apple, was diagnosed by Michael Forbes Wilcox, an autistic blogger. Wilcox writes that Jobs did 'think different', was often described as 'mercurial' and was creative. According to Wilcox, Jobs was clearly a genius; he and his kin 'push the human race forward'. The tentative diagnosis serves to explain focus, obsessive behaviours and a particular talent in a specific field and also associates Forbes Wilcox's own group (people with autism) with the 'genius' Jobs. Forbes Wilcox thus highlights autism as a condition to be proud of, one that confers strengths as well as challenges. Autism is cast as valuable and necessary for the progress of humanity. The green activist Greta Thunberg has similarly spoken of autism as her 'superpower'.[10]

Our work on this topic indicated that traits associated with autism could act *both* as strengths and challenges, depending on the circumstances.[11] Activists in the neurodiversity movement continue to cite strengths associated with autism, including high systemising skills, perfectionism and focus. All are potentially advantageous but only in the right circumstances. As noted in Chapter 4, the idea of psychological traits that bring strengths has underpinned arguments for neurodiversity as a valuable genetic variation.[12] The retrospective diagnosis of famous, talented, dead people reinforces the idea of autism as a source of self-worth and pride.

The reach of the autism diagnosis has been extrapolated so far back from the present day (at least in the UK) that it is now inferred in the ancient world via archaeological finds. A British academic identified autistic traits in the creators of Palaeolithic cave paintings because of their 'highly realistic detailed figurative representation, a focus on parts ... and a remarkable visual memory ... in common with autism'.[13] That autism is now able to stretch back thousands of years into prehistory and can be identified from artefacts, rather than in an embodied person, tells us how powerful the concept now is.

Retrospective diagnoses loop and influence the experts, health institutions and even people's understandings of themselves and each other (à la Hacking; see Figure 3.4). In the process of making a retrospective diagnosis, 'what counts' as autism is reformulated and extended to include new signs, for example 'detailed figurative representation', looping back to more imprecise lay understanding of 'what is autism' and spreading the use of the term.

The historian, Mathew Smith questions the idea of unchanging fixed categories in psychiatry, showing how diagnosing dead people as having attention deficit hyperactivity disorder (ADHD) has allowed psychiatry to frame it as a fixed entity, rooted in biology.[14] The diagnosis of the nineteenth-century fictional character *Johnny Head-In-Air* provides an example. Johnny was a character in an illustrated poem created by the German physician Heinrich Hoffmann in 1909. Despite being entirely fictional, Johnny is routinely cited in ADHD academic and research literature as an early account of a child with inattentive ADHD:[15, 16]

As he trudged along to school
It was always Johnny's rule
To be looking at the sky
And the clouds that floated by;
But what just before him lay,
In his way,
Johnny never thought about;
So that every one cried out—
'Look at little Johnny there,
Little Johnny Head-in-Air!'[17]

The function of Johnny's retrospective ADHD diagnosis is to show it is universal and has always been around. This may be particularly important for ADHD, because until recently, ADHD was a somewhat contested diagnosis in the public gaze, at least in the UK, as it has been a poster child for medicalisation.[18-20] This level of scepticism may prompt a defensive reaction from ADHD scientists who feel the subject of their enquiry is threatened. They therefore pick examples to demonstrate the universality, stability and unchanging nature of behaviours that, if seen today, would prompt an ADHD diagnosis. Johnny having ADHD legitimises ADHD as a category. ADHD is a theory that we use, but it is so useful in understanding the way nature works that we can almost call it real.

The same legitimising function sometimes applies to those retroactively claimed as having autism. According to Gernsbacher and his colleagues:[21]

> *The phenomenon of autism has existed most likely since the origins of human society. In retrospect, numerous historical figures … fit autism diagnostic criteria but were not so diagnosed in their day.*

The universality of autism through time can be equated with its biological, essential nature. If people with ADHD, and autism, have always existed, these categories are valid constructs. Retrospective diagnoses thus do meaningful work when operationalised as scientific fact, demonstrating that the diagnostic categories are carving nature at the joints.

Table 6.1 shows how Shea and colleagues – somewhat irreverently – retrospectively diagnosed the characters in AA Milne's *The House at Pooh Corner* (1928) in their article, 'Pathology in the Hundred Acre Wood: a neurodevelopmental perspective on A.A. Milne'.[22] Christopher Robin has also been rather ironically diagnosed by Cheryl Adams Richkoff[23] and MinJae Lee.[24] Humorous, and intended as holiday reading, Shea and colleagues use retrospective diagnosis to entertain us. But their diagnoses have stuck. The story of Winnie-the-Pooh's obsessive compulsive disorder (OCD), Roo's autism and Tigger's ADHD have been replicated in PowerPoint presentations at scientific conferences,[25] and teaching materials in schools, where the diagnoses of Pooh and his friends offer fluffy, non-threatening ways to introduce and talk about autism, ADHD and OCD to children.[26] In such contexts, however amusing, the diagnoses work to illustrate

Table 6.1 Retrospective diagnoses of characters in *Winnie-the-Pooh*

Winnie	ADHD (inattentive subtype), obsessive compulsive disorder (OCD)	Demonstrates impulsivity; for example, his poorly thought-out attempts to get honey; obsessive fixation on honey, which has contributed to his obesity
Kanga	Social anxiety disorder	Over-protective of her son, Roo; never lets Roo make his own decisions
Piglet	Generalised anxiety disorder	Anxious, blushing, flustered, stuttering; anxiety possibly stems from a crippled self-esteem
Eeyore	Depression/ dysthymia	Chronic negativism, low energy, never shows emotions such as joy or excitement
Tigger	ADHD	Impulsive sampling of unknown substances such as honey, haycorns and thistles; climbs tall trees and acts socially intrusively
Owl	Dyslexia	Gets his spelling wrong, with letters missing, swapped around or even written back to front; has trouble reading
Christopher Robin	Schizophrenia	Believes that all the characters in *Winnie-the-Pooh* are manifestations of his mood

Note: ADHD, attention deficit hyperactivity disorder.

the psychiatric categories as unwavering and firm. Their use in teaching materials demonstrates that diagnosable disorders of childhood have existed throughout history, since they were on AA Milne's mind, even though the disorders were unnamed until now. Thus the action of diagnosis has the function of reifying the diagnostic category. Pooh himself has been diagnosed by one autistic commentator as having autism.[27]

Childhood diagnoses are now firmly a part of children's landscape and language; consequently they should be addressed in the classroom. For me, this diagnostic reading diminishes the innocence and magic of the childhood of Christopher Robin. Childhood was once about wandering, playing with sticks and building with dirt.[28] Rereading via diagnosis means losing some of the romance. Piglet should probably be on Prozac, Adams Richkoff points out.[23]

The Pooh characters' diagnoses – 'Tigger has ADHD' – are knowledge objects, in social science terms.[29] Tigger's diagnosis now has its own life, used by generations of ADHD researchers to show ADHD has always been around. When they encounter hyperactivity, students learn to apply this knowledge to real-life phenomena and thus Tigger's diagnosis becomes an agent in creating knowledge about ADHD.[30]

What cannot immediately be seen in the classroom (because we are currently in the midst of the age of diagnosis) is that autism, ADHD and OCD diagnoses are unlikely to survive unchanged. Historians of the future looking at our era might examine Tigger and Roo's diagnoses as quirky artefacts that illustrate how people back in the old days thought about childhood behaviour and its classification as an attribute of a child. Retrospective diagnosis says more about the era, and the people doing the diagnosing, than it does about the person being diagnosed.

Svend Brinkmann has written about how mental health diagnoses comprise one of several possible explanatory frameworks for a person's difficulties.[31] Other frameworks include moral, existential, spiritual and political explanations. To illustrate his ideas, I drew Table 6.2 which gives a range of possible explanations for an adolescent working in a factory with very low mood.

Brinkmann argues diagnostic narratives often operate at the expense of other explanations. To take the political example above, many studies have shown that, as a person who is socio-economically disadvantaged is more likely to suffer very

Table 6.2 Some possible explanatory frames for low mood of adolescent working in factory

Frame	Very low mood due to	Reason	Action
Diagnostic	Depressive disorder	Biological imbalance	Take anti-depressant
Moral	Bad karma	Immoral actions of self	Behave better, atone
Political	Low pay, no prospects	Unjust society	Join a union
Spiritual	Ancestors angry	Spirits not at peace	Present offering, ritual
Existential	Inescapable part of life	Normal to suffer at adolescence	Do nothing, accept

low mood,[32] the argument is that taking an anti-depressant depoliticises and masks a social justice issue.[33]

People often draw on multiple narratives, but diagnosis is currently the go-to explanation for health troubles or mental difficulties, edging out other possibilities. Furthermore, each frame of understanding moderates how troubles are experienced. Anthropological studies have shown how women experience late middle age very differently in Japan to the USA.[34] US narratives revolve around menopause, whereas in more traditional families in Japan the end of menstruation is not considered significant; in contrast, late middle age is considered to be women's prime of life, and the term 'hot flush' did not exist until recently.[34] Although hot flushes are very often reported by women in the USA, they were rarely reported to be experienced by women in rural Japan.[34] Experience is thus mediated by how it is named or understood. Similarly, how a neurological difference is experienced is mediated by how it is named or understood and the sub-narratives this entails, as discussed in the previous chapter.

Child and adolescent psychiatrists like the excellent Tamsin Ford have positioned child mental health as everybody's business[35] through their work showing that disorders are highly prevalent in school-age children (estimates suggest one in nine children and adolescents were suffering from a probable mental disorder in the UK in 2017, a rise since 1999 with a further jump during the Lockdown in response to Covid-19, to one child in six in 2020[36]). Recognising the widespread nature of mental disorders destigmatises them, but such work also supplies an accessible language to think about children's troubles in a diagnostic, pathological framework. That psychiatric diagnostic language is an everyday occurrence in the classroom returns us to the Hundred Acre Wood: that Pooh has autism, and that autism has been lifted by a rising tide of culturally accessible diagnostic narratives.

None of this is to suggest Tigger does not have ADHD; his ADHD is not 'invalid'. All knowledge is valid, just situated;[37] valid in one situation, located in our time. The *Winnie-the-Pooh* diagnoses are well-intentioned ways of talking about difficult topics to children in an accessible way. They could also be seen as less benign, as establishing normal childhood ways of being as pathologies.[19] Instead of the wonderful thing about Tigger is him having boundless energy and being tons of fun, *circa* 2020, there is something amiss with him.

The autism lens

Rosenhan illustrated the diagnostic lens brilliantly in the 1970s' observational experiment 'On being sane in insane places'.[38] Rosenhan and his research team (all of whom were 'sane') applied for admissions to psychiatric institutions, complaining of hearing voices. All were admitted and most were diagnosed with schizophrenia. The team members documented how, during their hospitalisation, they reverted to behaving completely normally, yet many of their behaviours, actions and previous instances in their lives, however commonplace, were treated as pathological and illuminative of their schizophrenic state,[38] according to the notes taken by the institutional staff. This experiment underlines the tendency to interpret human social behaviour using a particular diagnostic lens.

What I would call the *autism lens* is a similar concept to the 'medical gaze'.[39] Medical trainees are taught to interpret bodies and behaviours in terms of their symptoms, producing the clinicians' expertise through their 'gaze'. This lens both actively constructs and renders pathology visible.[40] Once you recognise autism, you see it everywhere.[41]

In 2017, we enrolled four commentators on the Autism Diagnostic Observation Schedule (ADOS) professional training courses for clinicians and researchers, considered one of the best diagnostic tools to identify autism.[42] ADOS is a semi-structured assessment of communication, social interaction and play (or imaginative use of materials) for people suspected of having autism.[43] It is widely used in diagnostic centres in Europe and North America. Like many other psychiatric instruments used to measure disorder, ADOS is not free. Training in, and use of, the tool is a commercial enterprise. Only accredited researchers and clinicians are allowed on the training course, creating a limited number of professionals who, after qualifying, 'officially' become able to read and decode who has autism.[42] Two of the trainees we funded were autistic activist researchers, two were parents of children identified as being on the autism spectrum and one was a clinician noted for his critical perspective. The aim of ADOS is to observe autistic behaviour and repeatedly be able to rate it against a benchmark to a similar standard. In my reading of their accounts, ADOS training focused the autism lens. Training encouraged participants to interpret a child's videoed behaviour as autistic, whereas at least one initially read the behaviour as not.[42] The hope is that identification enables effective intervention that enables children to thrive.

On the other hand, autism can become a master status that over-rides and subsumes other identities and knowledge, trumping them in the eyes of others. An old friend once bemoaned how he wanted to be known as an artist rather than a 'black artist'. Art critics gave his ethnicity master status; it became the lens through which his every work was assessed. Katherine Runswick-Cole, a parent scholar, described how her child's autism label 'drowns out other stories that might be told about them'.[44] The autism lens of non-autistic others (engendered by the disclosure of her child's diagnosis) provides a discursive framework to 'story a life'. This applies to both the living and the dead.

Use of the lens can thus be a double-edged sword. More authority is given to those speaking in the field who have a diagnosis – diagnosis-as-asset, which can be deployed, can foster resilience,[45] but, at the same time, diagnosis, once disclosed, also undermines people's activities. The autistic academic, Melanie Yergeau, writes about her experience of the autism lens:

> *When my writing lacks transition, it is because I am autistic. When my fingers twirl in the air, fidgety and tangled in series of rubber bands, it is because I am*

autistic. When my eyes dart away or when my sentences grow long, it is because
I am autistic.[46]

Non-professionals who frequently develop an 'autism lens' include adults who
have a diagnosis of autism or an autistic identity or family members of those with
a diagnosis: that is, members of the autism community.[47] Adults diagnosed with
autism in adulthood, and parents of autistic children, often educate themselves
extensively about autism and develop a laser-like autism lens, a self-reported
ability to spot autism in others, hence some retrospective diagnosing of dead
people. I witnessed this first hand during my PhD research, when interviewing
parents whose children had received a diagnosis of autism.[48] Many of the parents
I interviewed discussed how autism had become visible everywhere since the
autism diagnosis had come on their radar:

> *We were sat the other day having a meal and there was a family with a quite*
> *young lad and he was chattering away to the parents and Harry and I just*
> *looked at each other and nodded. You kind of recognize it all the time. Watch*
> *things on television and say, 'That's Asperger's definitely' or autism (parent of*
> *diagnosed child).*[48]

Friends, relatives and casual strangers were now visible (to them) as autistic.
Occasionally, they approached others and offered the opinion that the other
might have autism.

The autism lens could be considered as a mechanism of social contagion –
the spread of information via social relations.[49] A key US study showed that
children were more likely to be diagnosed with autism if they lived near other
children diagnosed with autism spectrum disorder (ASD).[50] Tom Lister looked
at this process and identified two processes: more passive finding of autism
and more active seeking of autism by autistic adults.[41] He observed how the
lens led to 'lay diagnosis', which in turn could lead to self-identification and/
or a later referral to a clinic. This is perhaps one mechanism through which
social contagion takes place. The autism lens breeds more identification, more
visibility and more diagnosis; in short, another looping effect potentially contributing to autism's rise.

Does my dog have autism?

Retrospective diagnosis is just one way the autism label is applied outside the
doctors' clinic. It shows that autism has become an entity that exists in our minds
even without a living person to express it. Autism is now an idea separated and
dislocated from the human body, neatly illustrated by another practice that has
recently come to attention: diagnosing pets with very human disorders, a process
we dubbed 'anthropathography'.

There are websites and chatrooms dedicated to this practice. A US-based dog
care site, *Wag!*, provides a vivid example:

Can Dogs Get Autism?

Yes!

In some dogs who are suffering from autism, repetitive behavior such as incessant tail chasing may be one of the more predominant symptoms. It is possible for the dog to become aggressive during an episode and care should be taken when approaching. In others, the condition may result in withdrawn behavior and a lack of activity. In some dogs, the symptoms may be so mild you don't notice them but if you suspect your dog may have autism, you take him or her to your veterinarian for diagnosis.[51]

If humans display neurodiversity, no doubt so do other mammals. Dogs may or may not have similar types of neurodiversity. But diversity is not diagnosis! The diagnosis of autism in dogs relies on several assumptions:

- Autism is a category that can be transposed from humans to animals.
- The 'symptoms' listed have neurological origins and must be present from birth (indeed, *Wag!* states 'present from birth').
- Dog owners should look for neurological explanations for their pets' aberrant behaviour.

There are many obvious problems with such assumptions, not least that human social behaviour can be equated with that of dogs, that the linguistic anomalies characteristic of autism are absent, that repetitive behaviours are instigated by under-stimulation of captive animals (see Chapter 9) and there is apparently no developmental aspect to autism-in-dogs. The risk factors that precipitate autism-in-dogs, according to *Wag!* are probably a bitch's exposure to chemicals or inappropriate vaccinations during pregnancy.

The cardinal point is the transposition of autism from the human subject. Autism is transported wholesale as an idea. Autism-in-dogs illuminates the seductive power and reach of autism as a concept, strong enough to be dislocated from the human subject and survive the leap across the species boundary intact. Dislocation directly contradicts Sinclair's experience of autism as an integral aspect of himself, underpinned by his preference for the use of person-first language – 'autistic' rather than 'person with autism' – designed to prevent dislocation.[52]

Forms of diagnosis

The different ways to confer a diagnosis have multiplied. The *Exploring Diagnosis* team brought together many types of diagnosis beyond the standard medical diagnosis of the type one would receive in a clinic:

- Pre-diagnosis: identification of a person as being 'at risk' of being in a category
- Research diagnosis: identification of a person as having a category by researchers who measure symptoms and diagnose using a cut-off on a scale

- Self-diagnosis or self-identification: a person's identification of themselves as being in a category
- Lay diagnosis: a person without medical training identifies someone else as having the condition
- Pathography: identification of dead person as being in a category
- Paleopathography: diagnosis via artefacts or fragments from ancient civilisations
- Psychopathography: diagnosis of a dead person with a psychiatric condition
- Fictography (coined by Annemarie Jutel): a fictional person is identified as being in a category
- Anthropathography: a diagnostic category developed in humans is transferred to the diagnosis of another species (for example, diagnosing dogs).

Today, different forms of diagnosis explain much of the current deviance beyond obvious disease: diagnoses are given for people who are seen to be too determined, too related, too self-aware, too sad, too bouncy, too aggressive, too frequently drunk, too stupid, too repetitive and too aloof. As diagnosis became the best-known, most powerful and dominant way for clinicians to explain deviance from the statistical norm, diagnostic ways of understanding people and their troubles have spilled over from being the exclusive domain of clinicians, giving rise to different types of diagnosis. Parallel practices of diagnosis have arisen, motivated by different reasons, using medical diagnosis as a frame of reference but adapting it to the diagnosers' own ends. The process of diagnosis, whether by clinicians, lay people, family members or self-identifed, shapes the fabric of the diagnostic category as well as leading their interpretations of own or others' experience through its lens. In the modern context diagnosis, being named as this, or as that, also very often determines the pathway through care and through institutions. Eyal and colleagues suggest that autism was shaped in response to deinstitutionalisation and the need to intervene and group children in the therapeutic frame. So as well as determining a pathway through care, a diagnostic category may be shaped by the need to delineate a pathway.

If autism has become an entity that can be removed and transposed to unborn babies, dead people, fictional characters and dogs, what next? Autistic plants? Autistic machines? Insects with autism? This may not be as far-fetched as it sounds; ADHD genetics researchers have published world-leading studies on the genetics of ADHD using hyperactive fruit flies, a well-respected animal model.[53]

Although autism diagnosis has been rolled out to new populations, I do not want to suggest that neurological damage or differences are themselves 'artefactual'; they are not. Part I of this book has not been about there being more neurodevelopmental difference but about the extension of diagnosis to new populations. Post 1990, new sections of the human population; infants, intellectually able children, adults, and women have become eligible for autism diagnosis and inclusion of these new cohorts has directly increased the proportion of the people in our population with a diagnosis. Through this occurring, autism itself has been reshaped and reimagined, extending its reach even beyond the grave and beyond the human. As what is autism has shifted, so has what it means to be autistic, and the power of diagnosis to transform or story a life.

References

1. Jutel, A. & Russell, G. Past, Present and Imaginary: Pathography in all its Forms. *Rev.* (in development) (2020).
2. Foxhall, K. Making Modern Migraine Medieval: Men of Science, Hildegard of Bingen and the Life of a Retrospective Diagnosis. *Med. Hist.* **58**, 354–374 (2014).
3. Fitzgerald, M. *Autism and Creativity: Is There a Link Between Autism in Men and Exceptional Ability?* (Routledge, 2003).
4. Fitzgerald, M. *The Genesis of Artistic Creativity: Asperger's Syndrome and the Arts* (Jessica Kingsley Publishers, 2005).
5. Harley, N. Did Field Marshal Montgomery have Asperger's Syndrome? The Telegraph (22 May 2015).
6. Gillberg, C. Clinical and Neurobiological Aspects of Asperger Syndrome in Six Family Studies. In Autism and Asperger Syndrome (ed. Frith, U.) 122–146 (Cambridge University Press, 1991).
7. Fitzgerald, M. Did Ludwig Wittgenstein Have Asperger's Syndrome? *Eur. Child Adolesc. Psychiatry* **9**, 61–65 (2000).
8. Timms, C. Stark Raving Normal? The Psychologist. https://thepsychologist.bps.org.uk/volume-2018/february/stark-raving-normal (2018).
9. Elder, J. *Different Like Me: My Book of Autism Heroes* (Jessica Kingsley, 2005).
10. The Guardian. Greta Thunberg responds to Asperger's critics: 'It's a superpower'. www.theguardian.com/environment/2019/sep/02/greta-thunberg-responds-to-aspergers-critics-its-a-superpower (2019).
11. Russell, G. *et al.* Mapping the Autistic Advantage from the Accounts of Adults Diagnosed with Autism: A Qualitative Study. *Autism Adulthood* **1**, 124–133 (2019).
12. Singer, J. *NeuroDiversity: The Birth of an Idea* (Judy Singer, 2016).
13. Spikins, P. The Stone Age Origins of Autism. *Recent Adv. Autism Spectr. Disord. – Vol. II* (2013) doi:10.5772/53883.
14. Smith, M. *Hyperactive: A History of ADHD* (Reaktion Books, 2012).
15. Banaschewski, T. & Zuddas, A. *Oxford Textbook of Attention Deficit Hyperactivity Disorder* (Oxford University Press, 2018).
16. Faraone, S. V. *et al.* Attention-deficit/Hyperactivity Disorder. *Nat. Rev. Dis. Primer* **1**, 1–23 (2015).
17. Hoffmann, H. The English Struwwelpeter. *The British Library* www.bl.uk/collection-items/the-english-struwwelpeter-by-heinrich-hoffmann (1909).
18. Conrad, P. & Bergey, M. R. The Impending Globalization of ADHD: Notes on the Expansion and Growth of a Medicalized Disorder. *Soc. Sci. Med.* **122**, 31–43 (2014).
19. Conrad, P. & Potter, D. From Hyperactive Children to ADHD Adults: Observations on the Expansion of Medical Categories. *Soc. Probl.* **47**, 559–582 (2000).
20. Conrad, P. & Schneider, J. W. *Deviance and Medicalization: From Badness to Sickness* (Temple University Press, 1992).
21. Gernsbacher, M. A., Dawson, M. & Goldsmith, H. H. Three Reasons Not to Believe in an Autism Epidemic. *Curr. Dir. Psychol. Sci.* **14**, 55–58 (2005).
22. Shea, S. E., Gordon, K., Hawkins, A., Kawchuk, J. & Smith, D. Pathology in the Hundred Acre Wood: A Neurodevelopmental Perspective on A.A. Milne. *CMAJ* **163**, 1557–1559 (2000).

23. Adams Richkoff, C. The Characters in Winnie The Pooh All Represent Mental Illnesses. *Ranker* https://www.ranker.com/list/winnie-the-pooh-characters-represent-mental-illnesses/cheryl-adams-richkoff (2000).

24. Lee, M. Christopher Robin's Schizophrenia. *prezi.com* https://prezi.com/uz6hjp bkvii2/christopher-robins-schizophrenia/.

25. Humphrey, N. Are the kids alright? Exploring the intersection between education and mental health. 47. https://research.reading.ac.uk/andy/wp-content/uploads/sites/3/Neil-Humphrey-MHSchools17-Conference-Presentation-1.pdf.

26. Hetherington, K. Abnormality – Mental Health in Winnie the Pooh. *TES Resources* www.tes.com/teaching-resource/abnormality-mental-health-in-winnie-the-pooh-11412534.

27. Sinclair, J. Was Winnie-the-Pooh Created to Raise Awareness of Autism? *Autistic & Unapologetic* https://autisticandunapologetic.com/2018/07/28/was-winnie-the-pooh-created-to-raise-awareness-of-autism/ (2018).

28. Singh, I. & Wessely, S. Childhood: A Suitable Case for Treatment? *Lancet Psychiatry* **2**, 661–666 (2015).

29. Schrader, A. Responding to *Pfiesteria piscicida* (the Fish Killer): Phantomatic Ontologies, Indeterminacy, and Responsibility in Toxic Microbiology. *Soc. Stud. Sci.* **40**, 275–306 (2010).

30. Entwistle, N. & Marton, F. Knowledge Objects: Understandings Constituted Through Intensive Academic Study. *Br. J. Educ. Psychol.* **64**, 161–178 (1994).

31. Brinkmann, S. *Diagnostic Cultures: A Cultural Approach to the Pathologization of Modern Life* (Routledge, 2016).

32. Lorant, V. *et al.* Socioeconomic Inequalities in Depression: A Meta-Analysis. *Am. J. Epidemiol.* **157**, 98–112 (2003).

33. Brown, G. W. *Social Origins Of Depression: A Study of Psychiatric Disorder in Women* (eds. Brown, G. W. & Harris, T.) (Free Press, 1978).

34. Lock, M. & Kaufert, P. Menopause, Local Biologies, and Cultures of Aging. *Am. J. Hum. Biol. Off. J. Hum. Biol. Counc.* **13**, 494–504 (2001).

35. Ford, T., Hamilton, H., Meltzer, H. & Goodman, R. Child Mental Health is Everybody's Business: The Prevalence of Contact with Public Sector Services by Type of Disorder Among British School Children in a Three-Year Period. *Child Adolesc. Ment. Health* **12**, 13 (2007).

36. NHS Digital. Mental Health of Children and Young People in England. *NHS Digital* https://digital.nhs.uk/data-and-information/publications/statistical/mental-health-of-children-and-young-people-in-england (2019).

37. Haraway, D. Situated Knowledges: The Science Question in Feminism and the Privilege of Partial Perspective. *Fem. Stud.* **14**, 575–599 (1988).

38. Rosenhan, D. L. On Being Sane in Insane Places. *Science* **179**, 250–258 (1973).

39. Collins, H. & Evans, R. *Rethinking Expertise* (University of Chicago Press, 2007).

40. Mol, A. *The Body Multiple: Ontology in Medical Practice* (Duke University Press, 2003).

41. Lister, T. What's in a label? An exploration of how people acquire the label 'autistic' in adulthood and the consequences of doing so (University of Exeter, 2020).

42. Timimi, S., Milton, D., Bovell, V., Kapp, S. & Russell, G. Deconstructing Diagnosis: Four Commentaries on a Diagnostic Tool to Assess Individuals for Autism Spectrum Disorders. *Auton. Birm. Engl.* **1** (2019) AR26.

43. Lord, C., Risi, S. & Lambrecht, L. The Autism Diagnostic Observation Schedule-Generic; A Standard Measure of Social and Communication Deficits Associated With the Spectrum of Autism. *J Autism Dev Disord* **30**, 205–233 (2000).

44. Runswick-Cole, K. Understanding this Thing Called Autism. In *Rethinking Autism* (eds. Mallet, R., Timimi, S. & Runswick-Cole, K.) 19–30 (Jessica Kingsley Publishers, 2015).

45. Singh, I. A. Disorder of Anger and Aggression: Children's Perspectives on Attention Deficit/Hyperactivity Disorder in the UK. *Soc. Sci. Med. 1982* 73, 889–896 (2011).

46. Yergeau, M. Occupying Autism: Rhetoric, Involuntarity, and the Meaning of Autistic Lives. In *Occupying Disability: Critical Approaches to Community, Justice, and Decolonizing Disability* (eds. Block, P., Kasnitz, D., Nishida, A. & Pollard, N.) 83–95 (Springer Netherlands, 2016). doi:10.1007/978-94-017-9984-3_6.

47. Kenny, L. *et al.* Which Terms Should be Used to Describe Autism? Perspectives from the UK Autism Community. *Autism* 20, 442–462 (2015) doi:10.1177/1362361315588200.

48. Russell, G. & Norwich, B. Dilemmas, Diagnosis and De-stigmatization: Parental Perspectives on the Diagnosis of Autism Spectrum Disorders. *Clin. Child Psychol. Psychiatry* 17, 229–245 (2012).

49. Burt, R. S. Social Contagion and Innovation: Cohesion versus Structural Equivalence. *Am. J. Sociol.* 92, 1287–1335 (1987).

50. Liu, K., King, M. & Bearman, P. S. Social Influence and the Autism Epidemic. *Am. J. Sociol.* 115, 1387–1434 (2010).

51. Wag! Wag! https://wagwalking.com/wellness/can-dogs-get-autism (2019).

52. Sinclair, J. Why I Dislike 'Person First' Language. *Auton. Crit. J. Interdiscip. Autism Stud.* 1 (2013).

53. Rohde, P. D. *et al.* Testing Candidate Genes for Attention-deficit/Hyperactivity Disorder in Fruit Flies Using a High Throughput Assay for Complex Behavior. *Fly (Austin)* 10, 25–34 (2016).

Part II
'Real'

7   Epidemiology and lay epidemiology

Risk factors

In Chapter 1, we saw how population-based data have revealed an exponential increase in diagnosed autism in higher-income countries. This part examines whether there are plausible reasons for a 'real' increase; that is, a larger proportion of children and adults with autistic-type traits since 1990. If so, it is likely that changes in social and technological practices and environmental risk factors since 1990 have elicited more divergent neurodevelopment.

Talking about 'risk' positions autism as a problem; being 'at risk' of autism, as discussed in the previous part, means someone is more likely than an average person to be identified. 'Risk factor' is a term that comes from medical research, and brings with it an influence on how we view people's differences. Reading the literature on risk factors shows that only technical experts, trained epidemiologists, are able to quantify risks, that their studies originate from a medical standpoint, and they inevitably position the subject of the risk discourse (in this case autism), as being a problem that needs to be resolved. The idea of the 'risk factors' that precipitate autism and may have a role in increase of the proportion of people with autism traits, may be challenging for some in the neurodiversity movement, (see Figure I.2, Introduction) because the movement originated in resistance to parent-activism that positioned autism as distressing and problematic, parent-activism that strongly utilised this discourse of 'risk'. Environmental trigger theories were adopted by the hardcore faction in the this first wave of parent activists, whom may have seemed, to autistic self- advocates, to be intent on eliminating autistic people. Therefore the whole idea of risk and quantifying risk may be distasteful to leaders in this movement.

In the sections that follow, in order to review the evidence in the field, I have adopted the positivist framework, whilst hopefully, maintaining an awareness of the positions that various tribes have adopted, and why, utilising epidemiological language of 'risk factors'. Exposure to a 'risk factor', as reported in this part, increases the probability that a larger proportion of the exposed population will have autism. Some exposures have profound consequences for neural development and it is important to quantify them. Many risk factors have been studied, usually via epidemiological association studies that examine whether there are higher rates of autism in children who have been exposed to the factor of interest.

Vaccines and thimerosal have been the subject of controversy, yet have repeatedly been proven to have no link to autism.[1] But what of other environmental and social risk factors; can they plausibly explain a portion of the rise?

Plausibility check

For any environmental or social explanatory risk factor to be plausible, even as a very partial explanation, it must fulfil these four criteria:

1. Risk must have come into being or increased in the late modern age, circa 1990.
2. Risk must affect neurodevelopmental outcomes, especially eliciting autistic-type behaviours.
3. Risk must have been present in high-income countries.
4. Risk must have affected a significant proportion of the population.

Studies estimate the relative proportion of variance in outcomes of autism attributable to inherited risks, that is to familial (genetically inherited) factors. Autistic traits are heritable but the contribution of the environment is increasingly acknowledged. Up to half the liability for autism may be explained by environmental influences;[1] more recent studies attribute more variance to environmental factors, as discussed in Chapter 2.[2]

Studies that separate environmental from inherited influences often look at relatedness (siblings and especially twins) as a proxy measure of genetic inheritance, yet also consider the shared environmental and cultural influences of families. Genetic predispositions cannot easily be disentangled from environmental factors, even though researchers try to, because people with the same genetics normally share very similar pre- and post-natal environments. For example, monozygotic (identical) twins not only share the same genetic make-up but the same womb, the same environmental exposures during pregnancy and the same birth traumas. Although studying monozygotic twins who are separated at birth through adoption is the gold-standard approach for disentangling inheritance from environment, all these shared conditions still apply. Separated twins are likely to be placed in families from the same region, who will share cultural norms, including how autism is defined and recognised. In sibling and non-adoption studies, parenting style, school, experiences of childhood trauma, diet and local environmental exposures can usually be added to the list of shared environmental influences.

Another challenge to disentanglement is that, although a particular genetic profile predisposes an infant to atypical development, there is a complex interplay between genetic and environmental influences throughout development, leading to the expression of traits (perceptual, sensory, cognitive processing differences) as behaviours (Figure 7.1). Dichotomising the genetic and environmental contribution is therefore fraught. For example, exposure to an infection during pregnancy might trigger the expression of a foetal genetic mutation that subtly alters the child's neurodevelopment, perhaps increasing the chances of

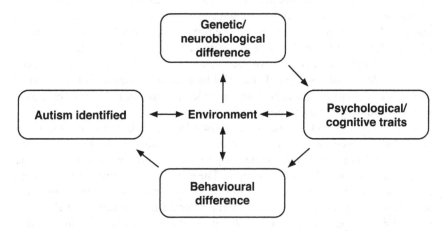

Figure 7.1 A model of identification in the clinic.

autism being identified in childhood. Without that particular genetic anomaly, the infection might have had no impact on the foetus. The interplay may be further complicated by multiple other environmental/genetic interactions, overlaid by the recognition, understanding, social context and diagnosis of autism, which is the outcome in many gene/environment studies.

Iodine is one example of a putative environmental risk factor. A severe lack of iodine in the diet during pregnancy can lead to stunting, cretinism and other neurodevelopmental problems in the child.[3] This is thought to be because the maternal thyroid hormone, which requires iodine, is crucial for the neurodevelopment of the foetus.[4] Our systematic review found no clear link between thyroid insufficiency in pregnancy and autism in the child, although there was an association between mothers' thyroid dysfunction and childhood indicators of intellectual disability.[5] There is no serious iodine deficiency in the diet of the mainstream population of the developed world, especially not since 1990. Therefore, iodine deficiency dose not pass the plausibility check and is an unlikely suspect for a risk factor to explain the rise in autism cases. But this is the type of environmental risk factor we might consider. To reiterate, for a risk factor to be a plausible contributor to a real rise in the number of neurodevelopmental diagnoses it must be: (1) recent (post-1990); (2) associated with autism; and (3) present in high-income countries where the trend is observed.

In the next chapter, I will review some candidate risk factors and assess their plausibility as triggers drawn from a study of what the wider autism community as opposed to the autistic community, have put forward.

Lay epidemiology

The first research study I conducted covered this topic. In 2004, Jean Golding, at that time the director of the Avon Longitudinal Study of Parents and Children

(ALSPAC), was awarded funding for an epidemiological study of environmental risk factors for autism. Her university put out a press release announcing the new research. Unsurprisingly, the press release prompted far-reaching media interest, with articles appearing in UK and international news outlets; Golding also gave several interviews to UK national radio and on local television. The publicity created a deluge of correspondence; Golding received around 100 unsolicited letters, e-mails and phone calls, many of which put forward theories about possible environmental triggers for autism.

By 2009, I was lucky to be co-supervised by Golding during my PhD. She suggested that I conduct an analysis of the correspondence (all of which she had carefully and conscientiously replied to) to see not only what correspondents were saying but how they were saying it. The unsolicited communications were a unique source of data, as they were not selected on the basis of any limiting criteria imposed by researchers. The content reflected the correspondents' views – very different from the 'co-produced' nature of data from traditional interview sources.[6] I re-contacted the correspondents to confirm they were happy to be included in the analysis, which we subsequently published.[7]

Almost all the correspondents were people who had close ties with autism. Some were parents with extensive experience caring for a child with autism, some were professionals with years in clinical practice and some were people with personal experience of autism, a group that Lorcan Kenny and colleagues loosely describe as 'the autism community'.[8] The correspondence broadly illustrated the strength of the correspondents' belief that the true incidence of autism is rising and that this was due to the use of modern technologies and to changing lifestyles. For example, a retired teacher wrote:

> *I have been amazed at the increased incidence of autism – and pondered about the causes as have other people … since I left in 1995 something has happened – an explosion. The autistic did not exist in quantity pre-1995 – so bearing in mind children enter schools at five years old – something changed around 1990 onwards. I don't think it can all be down to better detection of autism.*[7]

At the time, we used the term 'lay' to describe the correspondents but this does not quite capture their relationship with autism. As the sociologist Lindsay Prior has pointed out, the term 'lay-expert' is an oxymoron.[9] Together, these correspondents had enormous expertise. A few possessed traditional qualifications of scientific expertise, while others were non-traditional autism experts, having educated themselves extensively in autism literature; their expertise was not necessarily 'scientific' but none the less credible, valid and reflective of a view of expertise as fluency within a particular community.[10]

A handful of correspondents described how they had conducted ministudies to test their personal theories. They were experts but in a different way to trained epidemiologists; hybrids who could best be described as 'lay epidemiologists'.[11–13] In traditional epidemiology, the focus is on those causes which exert the largest effect; in lay epidemiology, the emphasis shifts to personal situations and draws on a wide range of sources. Lay epidemiology frequently shows the imprints of both the environmental justice movement and of critical epidemiology among trained epidemiologists.[13] The phenomenon has been discussed extensively by the sociologists Phil Brown[13] and Brian Wynne.[14] Wynne points out that the lay community has technical expertise; they know the everyday exposures and lifestyles that may be associated with any outcome. Brown describes lay epidemiology as a form of citizen science – not only an appropriation of professional methods but also a form of social movement, often through a politically mobilised group coming together around the goal of identifying and ameliorating environmental stressors and their relationship to health outcomes. Erin Brockovich was a lay epidemiologist; after witnessing the deteriorating health in the community, she discovered toxic chromium[6] was leaking into the groundwater sources in a Calfornian town, Hinkley. Her fight for social justice has been well documented and was the subject of an acclaimed Hollywood film.

My first study showed that lay epidemiology was an alternative form of expertise, harnessing information often drawn from insights hewn from the 'coal face' of autism. However, lay epidemiologists also co-opt the risk discourse to establish the causes of problems. Like traditional epidemiologists, being autistic is still positioned as something to be avoided, and risks to be mitigated; otherwise, there would be no reason to quantify risk.

Correspondents suggested more than 40 different environmental factors as potential reasons to explain autism's rise. The vast majority related to medical technologies or practices, modern environmental risk factors or our changing way of life (Table 7.1 divides these theories into three categories: medical technologies, environmental exposures and lifestyle or social changes). Association studies that examine whether there are higher rates of autism for children who have been exposed to a factor of interest rarely afford the autistic participants, or their parents, teachers or relatives, any agency. Paying attention to people with lived experience, and their ideas about risk, by giving the lay epidemiologists' questions and theories research time and credence may negate this.

The correspondence was unsolicited and there was so much of it! Its very bulk indicated a latent unease. Emotional investment, caring about autism, might seem antithetical to the objectivity of scientific enquiry. But in his book *Risk Society* Ulrich Beck warns against removing such human and emotional aspects from science.[15] Science should consider instead what is *culturally* significant, he says: 'Social movements raise questions that are not answered by the risk technicians at all and the technicians answer questions which miss the point of what was really asked and what feeds public anxiety'.[15]

The risks Beck describes are invisible but become known, or are made visible, through scientific measurement (that is, epidemiology). Science identifies, defines and responds to risks. Correspondents suggested that the technological applications of modern life could be risk factors for autism (defining it as a problem), requesting the science of epidemiology to confirm their theories (to enable a solution). Meanwhile, the correspondents remained anxious. Some had even changed their working practices. One correspondent, a dentist by trade, had taken to removing his patients' mercury amalgam fillings. Another, a midwife, wrote:

Table 7.1 Putative risk factors for autism taken from correspondents' theories

Medical technologies	
Pregnancy and birth	Ultrasound scans
	Baby-induced
	Early cord clamping/cord wrapped around baby's neck
	Respiratory distress at birth
	Caesarean section
	Birth trauma, low birth weight, pre-term
Related to drugs/toxins during pregnancy	Foetal stress due to medical intervention
	RhoGAM shots
	Contraceptive pill
	Steroids
	Antihistamines
	DES (to prevent miscarriage)
Related to vaccines	High levels of mercury due to dental fillings
	Time of day of vaccination
	Lack of aspiration when vaccine administered
	Measles, mumps and rubella vaccine
	Mercury due to thiomersal
	Vulnerability to injections when teething
	Polio vaccine
	Egg products in vaccines
	Pain of injection
	DPT vaccine/toxins
Changing lifestyle	
General	Working mother leads to stress during pregnancy
	Later motherhood
	Amount of alcohol drunk during pregnancy
	Time indoors
	Overstimulation by cot toys
	Too much television/computer/mobile phone
Related to modern diet	Lack of cod liver oil
	Food additives/aspartame
	Disaccharides and starches, sucrose
	Food preservatives
	Genetic origin of cow's milk due to intensive animal breeding
	Gluten in diet
Unavoidable environmental factors	
	Low-level radiation, e.g. computer monitors
	Carbon monoxide exposure
	Father works in nuclear power station/exposure to radioactivity
	Exposure to chemicals
	Living near mobile phone mast/exposure to low-level radiation
	Mould from indoor environments
	Air pollution/air quality
	Pollutants in water, pesticides
	Previous miscarriage or bleeding during pregnancy
	Dry birth (no amniotic fluid)
	Child being born after twins

Notes: DES, diethylstilbestrol; DPT, diphtheria, pertussis, tetanus.

There are those who believe there is a correlationship between the rise in autistic spectrum disorders and the practice of early umbilical cord clamping. ... As a midwife I find this very disturbing as this has been my practice and that of my colleagues. As a precautionary measure, I now leave the cord longer before cutting it, in order that the neonate might receive possibly 50% more of its blood supply from the placenta.

Such actions did not stem from 'misconceptions'. On the other hand, they were not 'correct', more that many merited further investigation. In the following chapter I review the evidence for one theory from each of the categories in Table 7.2, using the epidemiological language of 'risk factors'. The theories displayed logic and integrity, born from everyday exposure to autism in the context of their lives. Their intimate experiences with autism gave them a partial and located viewpoint, a form of situated knowledge.[16] The insights the correspondents provided came from varied sources of information, drawn both from personal and professional networks and the public arena.[11, 17, 18] This close, personal connection meant correspondents often had a viewpoint, sometimes accompanied by tremendous emotional investment in their own ideas, that traditional epidemiologists lacked.[7]

Separating autistic traits from diagnosis

These theories of putative risk factors for autism inspired the next ten years of my work. Following the lay epidemiology work and to help settle the issue of autism's diagnostic expansion versus more autism (or at least provide some partial evidence), we conducted a traditional epidemiological study that attempted to uncouple increase in diagnosis after 1990 from increase in traits. We examined population-based data to see whether the growth of diagnosis in children with autism over a ten-year period was mirrored by a parallel increase in the number of children with mild or severe traits of autism; in essence, whether the increased rate of diagnosis was due to an increase in the number of children with autism or an increase in recognition by autism diagnosis.[19]

Data measured many years apart are not always directly comparable; different studies use different measures of case ascertainment. To account for this, we analysed data from two consecutive UK cohorts that had like-for-like measures: ALSPAC, which follows around 14,000 children born in 1991 or 1992, and the Millennium Cohort Study (MCS) of 18,000 children born ten years later, in 2000 or 2001, which followed their cohorts from birth through childhood and into adulthood. Using data from both studies, we calculated the number of eight-year-old children with autism-type traits and the number with diagnosis in the late 1990s (the ALSPAC children), compared to the number of eight-year-olds with autism-type traits and the number with autism diagnosis in the late 2000s (the MCS children).

Had the levels of traits (as opposed to levels of diagnosis) increased? The important quality of these two datasets was that they both collected the same type of reports of autism diagnosis: how much eye contact children made, their empathy, their fondness of routines and details about their communication abilities.[20] Despite being ten years apart, both studies used the same measures to gather some of their information. We found eight common measures, taken from teacher and parent reports, that were highly associated with the autism diagnosis, including poor communication, being less able to sustain peer relationships, being afraid of new situations and not being able to share easily or empathise well with other children. We fused these into a rough measure of autistic traits.

Inevitably, some data were missing, as not all families and schools enrolled in the cohort studies had completed the reports. Because of this, we analysed data where more than half the scores were present, which provided a large sample of approximately 16,000 children. The merged traits produced a composite score for each child, a coarse measure of how 'autistic' children were. We called this 'the composite autism-type traits score' (CATS).

The CATS were actually fairly normally distributed in the population of children as a whole and gave us the approximate distribution of autism traits in the whole population already illustrated in Figure I.5 in the Introduction. Most children fell into the mid-range. Of children who had an autism diagnosis at eight years old, 70% fell into the top 5% of scores. We also defined a threshold for 'severe CATS', defined as the top 1% of CATS. This told us that, although not a perfect measure of autism traits, CATS was a reasonable approximation, and probably the best we could hope for given the limitations of the two datasets.

Our hypothesis was consistent with the 'artefactual' explanation of the rise in autism diagnosis: that a larger proportion of children would be diagnosed in the later cohort but there would be no parallel increase in the proportion of children with autism-type traits. As predicted, there was a sharp rise in autism diagnosis between the two cohorts. In 1998, about 1.1% of eight-year-olds reportedly had an autism diagnosis, compared to 1.7% in 2008. Autism diagnosis rates had increased dramatically in the ten-year gap. As we had anticipated, in the two groups of eight-year-olds with severe CATs, there was no parallel jump in numbers; the proportion of children who had severe traits remained stable despite increased diagnosis.

Our findings were not entirely what we expected. Intruigingly, the proportion of children with milder traits (the 5% threshold) had increased in MCS compared to the proportion in ALSPAC ten years earlier, in tandem with the proportion with a diagnosis (Figure 7.2).

The study was an attempt to answer a big question. However, it suffered from several limitations, which reviewers were quick to point out when the study was submitted for publication. Some reviewers were very strong in their criticism of the paper, although others liked it. One problem was that the two cohorts were quite different in their make-up, geographical distribution and comparability. CATS was not a validated autism score, so some reviewers questioned the measure we used. It was hard to find a home for the work; it travelled to several high-impact journals, including the *British Medical Journal* (*BMJ*) before it eventually settled into a relatively low-impact journal, *BJPsych Open*.[19]

As the paper travelled through various journals and accrued rejections, I began to lose faith in the work but, at the same time, I wondered if reviewers from the

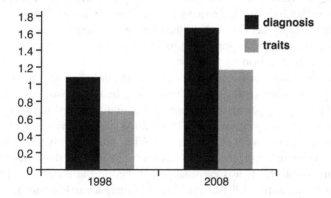

Figure 7.2 Change in mild traits and diagnosis in eight-year-olds in 1998 (Avon Longitudinal Study of Parents And Children (ALSPAC)) compared to 2008 (Millennium Cohort Study (MCS)) (top 5% composite autism-type traits score (CATS)).

medical establishment might not like the tentative conclusion that milder autism traits *might* have increased in the general population, being worried it might fan the flames of the anti-vaccine 'believers'. For example, on the manuscript's journey to its final destination, one anonymous reviewer for *Journal of the American Academy of Child and Adolescent Psychiatry* commented:

> *Child and adolescent psychiatrists have been telling the public for decades that vaccines, for example, do not substantially increase the rates of autism. We have a professional obligation to anticipate how our literature may be perceived by the public and what our publication will be communicating. This article could be interpreted by those who are strong proponents of 'environmental' autism theories (vaccines, chelation therapy, etc.) as evidence that their claim is true.*

One reading of this review, from a sociological standpoint, is that the reviewer indicates is there is only one approved way to have 'professional obligations' and those obligations appear to be mostly self-serving, by which I mean stabilising the authority of the discipline. This is the power relation: the voices within (such as that of the peer reviewer) have the authority. The profession/discipline's agency is undermined by any marginal inside voices that might be taken as support for voices on the outside who might challenge the disciplinary position.

As an epidemiologist, I could point out that the work was perhaps fundamentally methodologically flawed and no speculation could be based on the results. But were the methods *too* flawed to support a discussion that even raised the possibility of a real rise? Had a stronger methodological approach or data been employed, stronger conclusions would have been warranted. Was it, in fact, a question of good scientific practice? Although both positions are valid, this illuminates the tension between being both a quantiatively minded epidemiologist and a qualitatively minded social scientist. This is an issue of interdisciplinarity, that language and practices of each discipline are constrained and limit the possibilities of thought and expression, a topic I return to with reference to risk discourse in the next section.

At the same time as we submitted our work, unbeknownst to us, a similar article was submitted to the *BMJ*. This article, based on Swedish data, took a very similar tack, comparing time trends in autism diagnosis with parents' reports of autism symptoms over ten years (1993–2002). The sensitivity and specificity of the reported measure were similar to CATS. The Swedish article concluded that, although rates of diagnosis of autism were increasing, there was no parallel increase in symptoms. It was eventually published in the *BMJ* and had an enormous international reach.[21] But even this high-impact article had its limits: the parent-reported measure of autism was based on a very small sub-set of the data. Only 12 children were rated as having more severe symptoms of autism when the symptoms were first measured and 13 at the close. Nevertheless, this Swedish study had a larger overall sample size, like-for-like measures and many more time points than our study.

No study is without its limitations. There are inherent methodological challenges to all longitudinal, cross-cohort studies: sample sizes, comparable cohorts, comparable forms of measurement and so on. 'Exercise caution in interpretation' is the message. After multiple apprehensive reviews of our study, and some positive ones, I rewrote the concluding section of our article, abandoning any suggestion that autism might *really* be on the rise, as we were unable to provide any truly conclusive answers to the real-versus-artefactual debate. Instead, we reported our findings as a probable artefact of increased reporting of traits by parents and teachers, whose ratings primarily made up the CATS. The article concluded that the jump in the number of children with milder traits was likely to be as artefactual as the increase in diagnosis. This observed rise, I wrote, was probably due to teachers' and parents' increasing *identification* of autistic-type childhood behaviours.[19] Unfortunately, this unintentionally threw the objectivity of the parent-reported symptoms in the yet-to-be-published *BMJ* paper into question.

Despite this experience, I still think it is important to at least hold open the *possibility* that neurodevelopmental issues are on the increase in the population at large, however slightly. The observed shift might not be entirely 'artefactual'. If this is the case, a proportion of the increase, however small, is likely to be underpinned by relatively new social or medical practices like those highlighted by our lay epidemiologists.

Covid-19 and the discourse of risk

The empirical studies discussed in this part all operationalise the concept of risk as unproblematic, and this is how I have used the construct. As discussed above, the concept of risk is not benign but positions autism as something to be avoided, as a 'disrupted' neurodevelopment. Risk studies discursively position autism as a threatening entity; for this reason they may be objectionable to some radicals in the neurodiversity movement. The justification for the study of risk factors for autism is often that, by quantifying risks, autism and other neurodevelopmental outcomes can be avoided by mitigating the risk, that is, by intervention through policy or practice. Before considering the plausibility of risk factors for autism, it is worth considering Beck's, and other social theorists, contributions to thinking about the 'discourse of risk'.

The outbreak of Covid-19 provides a demonstration of how risk has come to dominate political action and governance, both through risk calculation (of something that may or may not happen in the future) and the mitigation of risk, an endeavour Beck sees as characteristic of our late modern age. Beck's work discusses how previously invisible risks are rendered visible by technical experts (in the case of Covid-19, the risks posed were rendered visible by epidemiologists and modellers) and how these definitions of risk overtly direct the political governance of society. Science not only defines the risk or the problem but scientific or technical experts also provide the solution (for example, a vaccine).

The result is that power becomes concentrated in the hands of a small cabal of experts who are qualified to assess the risk and recommend forms of mitigation. Decision making is removed from the population, which is ill qualified either to define risk or provide the best aversion strategy. Hence, the majority is left both enforcing the strategy and mitigating for the damage of the strategy itself. The lockdown in response to Covid-19 was a population-level medical intervention in response to a medically defined risk calculation. This is the 'discourse of risk', in which risk to life is discussed and dissected and action or intervention is demanded. Beck's work has further been used to dissect the threat of 'weapons of mass destruction' defined by a small number of experts in intelligence agencies before the Iraq War, antibiotic resistance and the terrorist threat.[22] For Covid-19, risk is the dominant discourse and Beck's work seems highly salient. Albeit, unlike the weapons, Covid-19 is very real.

Michel Foucault had quite a different notion of risk. In his book *Discipline and Punish,* he describes the difference between normal and pathological states but his attention is on the normalising gaze that regulates the way we behave and present ourselves in public and in our community and how this is linked to a moralising discourse.[23] Foucault's early work defines biopower as the form of power that controls human bodies, interaction and populations, which not only flows hierarchically from above to below (judges to accused, monarchs to subjects) as in the pre-modern era but is also wielded through surveillance – community surveillance and, in particular, self-surveillance.[24] Power circulates and is employed through a net-like organisation. People police each other and police their own behaviour; the action and stances they take are shaped by discipline and self-control. Foucault's ideas about surveillance seem highly relevant to the community policing during the Covid-19 lockdowns, although his impersonal concept of power does not mean it is held equally. Power still acts to keep some in subservient roles and others in control. To Foucault, discourse is the practice that shapes the objects of knowledge of which we speak: beliefs, ideas, concepts, language together make up a system of representation that organises our relation to reality.

Discourses such as those surrounding Covid-19, and autism, do not simply describe reality but, according to Foucault, shape, and teach us, how we see reality, so there are only certain ways in which we are able to talk about a topic. The autistic activist, Nick Walker, calls discourse of the risk underlying autism science the 'pathology paradigm'.[25] In this, the risk discourse contains the underlying assumption that population-wide screening, defining risk and intervening are desirable, even if currently impractical, underpinned by the discourse that an undesireable outcome should be eliminated, when possible.

The limited palette of language for talking about an outcome is exacerbated by the media's propagation of a risk discourse that highlights threats. In early 2020, in both the UK and the USA, commentators and politicians drew on metaphors of 'battle' and 'war' to motivate the common moral endeavour to protect the vulnerable from Covid. In the UK, daily counts of the deaths from Covid-19 were widely reported during the worst of the outbreak (reminiscent of the death toll of *The Hunger Games*[26]). Yet there was an excess of deaths above and beyond the number expected for the time of year that were not due to Covid-19 although there were not as many of them, these lives were equally important, yet they were not subject to the same daily roll call. These excess deaths could be attributed to the effects of lockdown, such as a reluctance to seek care, delays in receiving medical treatment, isolation or unidentified Covid-19. But it was the risk of death from confirmed Covid-19 that was highlighted, breeding anxiety and promoting surveillance by accentuating the danger of death both for those at high risk (mainly vulnerable elderly people with existing health problems) and those at very low risk (young, healthy people) to ensure compliance to new behavioural norms and foster self-and community surveillance to uphold them. At the time of writing, Covid-19 has become more normalised and the discourse has shifted as the surveillance role that the population occupies is less heightened.

The 'war' against Covid-19 is an example of how language has contributed to risk discourse. It is reminiscent of the proliferation of other discourses of risk, for example, the 'obesity epidemic' discourse, in which the media act as amplifiers and moralisers.[27] In contrast, the 'autism epidemic' is an unorthodox and highly contested phrase, because of the unwanted mobilisation around its rise, yet autism is still associated with risk and being at risk. The positioning of autism as something to be dreaded and eliminated has motivated activism in the autistic rights and neurodiversity movement, as discussed in Chapter 4.

The Covid-19 lockdowns in Europe, the USA and elsewhere, then, relied on community control, self-policing and surveillance to create a 'new normal'. For Foucault, writing decades ago, the social institutions of school, prisons, hospital and so on are sites of surveillance that act as 'a means of control and method of domination'.[23] Institutional mechanisms, such as exams, medical training and qualification, link 'a certain type of the formation of knowledge' to 'a certain form of the exercise of power'.[23] Thus, in Foucauldian terms, epidemiological expertise and epidemiological modelling create knowledge of Covid-19 and its predicted transmission. To legitimise interventions, politicians defer to epidemiological experts. The population surrenders its power to determine the best course of action and patients surrender themselves to treatment by clinicians who become war heroes.

The potential *risks* of long-term lockdown formed another, alternative discourse of risk, based on a different outcome to risk of loss of life. What was at risk was not merely damage to the economy but the exacerbation of inequalities across the divides that define the lines of power: across gender, race and class. Lockdowns hit the disadvantaged hardest, exacerbating inequality and risking public health, as poverty is the biggest killer of all. For many people in the 'gig economy', who live a hand-to-mouth existence, it was not possible to earn money during the lockdown. People outside the system were not eligible for state support. Social distancing was hard for more disadvantaged people who lived in crowded urban areas and who needed public transport to get to work. Globally, domestic violence against women (and children), who perhaps relied on frustrated husbands who suddenly had little or no income, increased during lockdowns. Women and members of ethnic minorities predominated in low-paid caring roles or in caring for elderly relatives, making them susceptible to infection. Members of ethnic minorities, as well as suffering higher death rates, were disproportionately represented in the key workers' groups, often in low-paid and insecure jobs. Education happened in a much more haphazard way for the poorest than the richest. Women carried the brunt of childcare and children's education in the newly pertinent domestic sphere.

The mechanisms of democracy and free speech were also 'at risk'. In some countries, the need for mass intervention of social distancing was used to suppress #BlackLivesMatter rallies after the death of George Floyd. Hungary fell victim to a new regime that took sweeping new powers to rule by decree; the Covid-19 pandemic and the measures needed to control it were used to justify the extension of state control, such as a new law proposing the end of legal gender recognition for transgender people. Journalists who opposed the government were unable to report the pandemic accurately and faced gaol for unauthorised reporting.[28] Márton Békés, a pro-government magazine editor, commented on Hungarian television that, as Hungary was now in a 'war situation', government control was necessary and opposition media outlets who drew attention to widening inequalities were 'openly rooting for the virus'.[28] Covid-19 interventions and risk discourse were used to justify the concentration of power and suppression of free speech.

A competing and parallel risk discourse provoked by the Covid-19 pandemic was, and is, the discourse of planetary risk. Environmentalists pleaded that the focus should remain on planetary health; that climate change and the health of the planet were the big picture. The lockdowns saw widespread changes in human behaviour and encouraged companies to alter their everyday operations. Millions of employees worked at home, reducing congestion, improving air quality and lowering levels of particulate air pollution. A Tweet proclaiming 'Coronavirus is Earth's vaccine. We're the virus' had, at the time of writing, received more than 500,000 likes and 80,000 retweets, some calling for permanent limits on human movement and industry.[29] Similar rejoicings accompanied the huge decline in aviation and the collapse of oil prices. The environmental lobby want us to learn the lessons of lockdown, advocating for some changes, such as home working and the demise of extensive tourism, to become more permanent.

Risk calculation is a thoroughly uncertain endeavour and the competing discourses swirling around Covid-19 illustrate there are different points of view on what should be deemed an important outcome, what is at risk, what should be mitigated for and what considered a bad outcome. The upshot of action to mitigate or control risk is that more and different risks spring up. Beck writes that risk society:

> *draws attention to the limited controllability of the dangers we have created for ourselves. The main question is how to take decisions under conditions of manufactured uncertainty, where not only is the knowledge base incomplete but more and better knowledge often means more uncertainty.*[30]

This is worth considering in autism discourse: the risk of what? Many measures are considered and tested and their outcomes are modelled. Increasingly, scholars have argued that reducing autism itself is less important than improving quality of life and well-being.[31]

Autism has its own discourse of risk. That is, autism is positioned as an outcome to be avoided. As with other risks, uncertainty in the calculation of risk is inherent in the studies of risk factors for autism. In the next chapter I will describe work that considers the risk of having autism, as measured by research scales (measuring autistic behavioural traits) and/ or diagnosis.

References

1. Modabbernia, A., Velthorst, E. & Reichenberg, A. Environmental Risk Factors for Autism: An Evidence-based Review of Systematic Reviews and Meta-analyses. *Mol. Autism* **8**, 13 (2017).
2. Sandin, S. *et al.* The Familial Risk of Autism. *JAMA* **311**, 1770–1777 (2014).
3. Pearce, E. N., Lazarus, J. H., Moreno-Reyes, R. & Zimmermann, M. B. Consequences of Iodine Deficiency and Excess in Pregnant Women: An Overview of Current Knowns and Unknowns. *Am. J. Clin. Nutr.* **104**, 918S–923S (2016).
4. Escobar, G. M. de, Obregón, M. J. & Rey, F. E. del. Iodine Deficiency and Brain Development in the First Half of Pregnancy. *Public Health Nutr.* **10**, 1554–1570 (2007).
5. Thompson, W. *et al.* Maternal Thyroid Hormone Insufficiency During Pregnancy and Risk of Neurodevelopmental Disorders in Offspring: A Systematic Review and Meta-analysis. *Clin. Endocrinol. (Oxf.)* **88**, 575–584 (2018).
6. Hammersley, M. & Atkinson, P. *Ethnography: Principles in Practice.* (Routledge, 1994).
7. Russell, G. & Kelly, S. Looking Beyond Risk: A Study of Lay Epidemiology of Childhood Disorders. *Health Risk Soc.* **13**, 129 (2011).
8. Kenny, L. *et al.* Which Terms Should be Used to Describe Autism? Perspectives from the UK Autism Community. *Autism* **20**, 442–462 (2015) doi:10.1177/1362361315588200.

9. Prior, L. Belief, Knowledge and Expertise: The Emergence of the Lay Expert in Medical Sociology. *Sociol. Health Illn.* **25**, 41–57 (2003).

10. Collins, H. & Evans, R. *Rethinking Expertise* (University of Chicago Press, 2007).

11. Frankel, S., Davison, C. & Smith, G. D. Lay Epidemiology and the Rationality of Responses to Health Education. *Br. J. Gen. Pract.* 41(351): 428–430.

12. Allmark, P. & Tod, A. How Should Public Health Professionals Engage with Lay Epidemiology? *J. Med. Ethics* **32**, 460–463 (2006).

13. Brown, P. Popular Epidemiology Revisited. *Curr. Sociol.* **45**, 137–156 (1997).

14. Wynne, B. May the Sheep Safely Graze? A Reflexive View of the Expert–lay Knowledge Divide. In *Risk, Environment and Modernity* (eds. Lash, S., Szerszynski, B. & Wynne, B.) 44–83 (Sage, 1996).

15. Beck, U. *Risk Society: Towards a New Modernity* (Sage, 1992).

16. Haraway, D. Situated Knowledges: The Science Question in Feminism and the Privilege of Partial Perspective. *Fem. Stud.* **14**, 575–599 (1988).

17. Davison, C., Smith, G. D. & Frankel, S. Lay Epidemiology and the Prevention Paradox: The Implications of Coronary Candidacy for Health Education. *Sociol. Health Illn.* **13**, 1–19 (1991).

18. Watterson, A. Whither Lay Epidemiology in UK Public Health Policy and Practice? Some Reflections on Occupational and Environmental Health Opportunities. *J. Public Health* **16**, 270–274 (1994).

19. Russell, G., Collishaw, S., Golding, J., Kelly, S. E. & Ford, T. Changes in Diagnosis Rates and Behavioural Traits of Autism Spectrum Disorders Over Time. *BJPsych Open* 1(2), 110–115 (2015). doi:10.1192/bjpo.bp.115.000976.

20. Steer, C. D., Golding, J. & Bolton, P. F. Traits Contributing to the Autistic Spectrum. *PLoS One* **5**, e12633 (2010).

21. Lundström, S., Reichenberg, A., Anckarsäter, H., Lichtenstein, P. & Gillberg, C. Autism Phenotype Versus Registered Diagnosis in Swedish Children: Prevalence Trends Over 10 Years in General Population Samples. *BMJ* **350** 0959–8138 (2015).

22. Spence, K. World Risk Society and War Against Terror. *Polit. Stud.* **53**, 284–302 (2005).

23. Foucault, M. *Discipline and Punish: The Birth of the Prison* (Vintage, 1995).

24. Sawicki, J. *Disciplining Foucault: Feminism, Power, and the Body* (Routledge, 1991).

25. Walker, N. Autism and the Pathology Paradigm. https://neurocosmopolitanism.com/autism-and-the-pathology-paradigm/ (2016).

26. Collins, S. *The Hunger Games* (Scholastic, 2009).

27. Monaghan, L. F., Rich, E. & Bombak, A. E. Media, 'Fat Panic' and Public Pedagogy: Mapping Contested Terrain. *Sociol. Compass* **13**, e12651 (2019).

28. Walker, S. Hungarian Journalists Fear Coronavirus Law may be Used to Jail Them. *The Guardian* (3 April 2020).

29. Hayes, J. Some Greens Rejoice Over Environmental Effects of COVID-19 Restrictions. www.mackinac.org/some-greens-rejoice-over-environmental-effects-of-covid-19-restrictions (2020).

30. Beck, U. *World Risk Society* (Polity Press, 1999).

31. Rodogno, R., Krause-Jensen, K. & Ashcroft, R. E. 'Autism and the Good Life': A New Approach to the Study of Well-being. *J. Med. Ethics* **42**, 401–408 (2016).

8 Risks during conception, pregnancy and birth

Risk factors

When considering risk factors for autism, it is not sensible to consider autism as one discrete diagnosable entity because the same types of risks are likely to underpin multiple neurodevelopmental traits that cut across different categories of disorder.[1-10] The co-occurrence of autism with attention deficit hyperactivity disorder (ADHD) is around 30%, the overlap of autism and intellectual disabilities is in the range of 50% and the co-occurrence with epilepsy roughly 20%.[11] Internalising disorders, such as anxiety and depression, also frequently co-occur with autism, although this may be a result of exclusion, rejection and bullying.[12] A family history of autism is, of course, a risk factor but so are other parental psychiatric disorders, clouding the boundaries between co-inherited traits of various disorders.[13] Despite this, journals and disciplines are often organised around diagnostic categories and epidemiologists examining risk factors often write about risk predicting different diagnostic categories (autism, ADHD, etc.). Diagnostic categories may not always cut nature at the joints but are how epidemiologists, publishing houses and their readers and clinicians have historically structured, communicated and understood their work on risk.

In this chapter, I will review studies of factors that predict having both autism and broader neurodevelopmental disorders and summarise the evidence on three potential early risk factors for autism. I have conducted three brief reviews, one for each candidate risk, each a contender put forward by the lay epidemiologists of the previous chapter: older parenthood, pre-term birth and air pollution.[14] Of course, this is not a comprehensive review of all the possible risk factors for autism; rather, these examples allow for some consideration of how social shifts, new aspects of the built environment and changing medical practice may, or may not, be plausible as triggers accounting for a portion of the observed rise.

Older parenthood

The time trend

Since 1990, in high-income countries, the average age at which women give birth has steadily increased. Figure 8.1 shows the average age of mothers in the UK

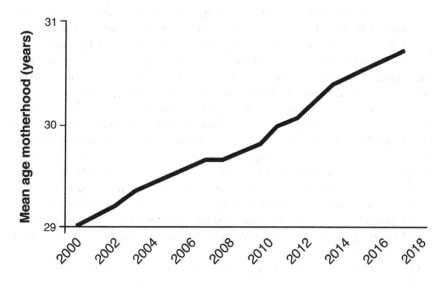

Figure 8.1 Time trend to older motherhood. UK data from the Office for National Statistics.

from 2000 to 2018. In Germany, the UK and France, mothers' average age at the birth of their first child is now more than 30; in Sweden, where gender equality is high, more than a quarter of women have children after the age of 35.

The picture is moderated by the strong correlation between the mother's age at childbirth and her education level.[15] Well-educated women more often delay childbirth than do less-educated women. On average, having a university degree defers the age of starting a family by seven years.[15] Consequently, there has been a sharp increase in women over 35 (and over 40) having babies. This is probably because well-educated women are more often financially independent and have access to fertility treatment (and contraceptives) and thus are able to defer pregnancy in favour of their career, maximising their earning potential and gaining time to undertake other pursuits. The demographic trend in fathers' age follows a similar trajectory. Since 1970, the average age of first-time fathers has increased annually in all the 23 Organisation for Economic Co-operation and Development (OECD) countries for which data are available.[16] The rise in second marriages for men, sometimes to women much younger than themselves, can also mean they become a father at a more advanced age.

Evidence of association

Numerous studies, including one of ours, have identified a link between older motherhood, and/or older fatherhood, and offspring with autism, although the evidence of the link with older motherhood is less conclusive than that with older fathers.[17] One problem is that some studies, including our own, do not control for the interaction with the other parent's age. One study of more than a million children in Denmark avoided this problem.[18] This study found an association, independent of the other parent's age, between both maternal and paternal age and their child's later autism diagnosis. Intriguingly, the effect for fathers was greatest when mothers were less than 35 years old, and *vice versa* for mothers. Interestingly, there is evidence that both autism and ADHD are more likely outcomes for children of very young mothers as well as older mothers.[19]

A second problem in assessing the impact of parental age comes from pooling data across consecutive cohorts, sometimes from cohorts where children were born more than 20 years apart, which tends to over-estimate risk because the incidence of autism diagnosis is rising.[20] Another large study, which examined data from more than four million children in California born between 1992 and 2000, took this into account.[20] This study found an increased risk of having a child with autism in mothers of more than 40 years old and a parallel, but limited, effect of the father's age. A Swedish study, including more than 400,000 children, found the effect of age on the risk of having a child with autism was stronger for mothers than fathers.[21]

A further Scandinavian study, again using Swedish data, this time of more than a million people, concluded fathers' age independently determined the increased risk, over and above other risks, for autism, including inherited traits (which they assessed via controlling for risk of autism in the fathers' other children).[22] The same group conducted a systematic review that meta-analysed data from 12 studies on the same topic.[23] This found evidence for both maternal and paternal age effects, estimating that the risk of having an autistic child increases by 18% for every ten years' increase in the mother's age, with a 21% rise in risk for every ten years' worth of deferred fatherhood. Findings were similar in an updated review.[24] Parental age at birth was more strongly associated with autism plus intellectual disability (ID) than for autism without ID. The paternal age effect extends to conditions beyond autism, with studies showing late fatherhood is linked to schizophrenia, as well as to dyslexia, reduced intelligence[25] and ADHD[19] in their offspring. Older maternal age has been associated with Down's syndrome[26] and childhood cancer.[27]

However, research documenting an increased risk of autism, or indeed the increased risk of any other condition, usually neglects the potential *benefits* of being born to late-producing, well-educated parents. Being born to older parents is advantageous in some ways, probably because of the association with high education and high socio-economic status.[16] Improved language, social and emotional health, and academic attainment have been associated with later motherhood, for example.[28]

Explanations of association – see Figure 8.2

The most prominent hypothesis in the literature, shown in Figure 8.2 as pathway (i), is that spontaneous genetic mutations (known as *de novo* mutations), which occur more often in older parents' sperm and eggs, are responsible for increased

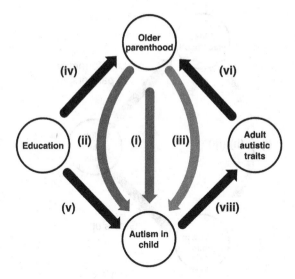

(i) *De novo* mutations
(ii) Pregnancy and birth complications (mother only)
(iii) Epigenetic accumulation
(iv) Delayed parenting for career
(v) Autism awareness: increased identification
(vi) Late formation of partnerships
(viii) Inherited traits

Figure 8.2 Schematic of possible explanatory pathways for association.

risk of disrupted neurodevelopment. Studies have found higher rates of *de novo* mutations in autistic children, with some variants common between autism and ID, especially copy number variants, in which chunks of chromosome are accidentally replicated, deleted, inverted or translocated during cell division.[29, 30] Copy number variants at specific chromosomal locations are thought to have a role in autism susceptibility. The *de novo* mechanism is consistent with the observation that a child with autism who has an older father is likely to be the father's only child with autism.[31] However, in the Danish study,[18] having both an older mother and an older father conferred no cumulative risk, which we would expect if the increased risk were due to new mutations.

Another suggested mechanism linking older motherhood to autism (Figure 8.2, pathway ii) is that older mothers are more likely to experience birth complications, including higher rates of birth by Caesarean section, premature birth and low birth weight,[32] which have been associated with childhood autism, ID and neuro-disability.[33] The impact of advanced maternal age on birth weight has apparently decreased over time as peri-natal services have improved,

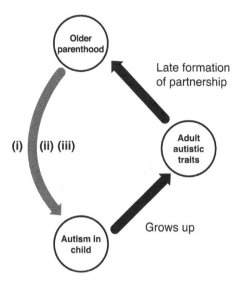

Figure 8.3 Putative looping effect from older parenting.

suggesting some effects of maternal age on child outcomes are not absolute but depend on the circumstances of the pregnancy and the services available.[33, 34]

Another possible pathway is the contribution of epigenetic changes (Figure 8.2, pathway iii). Distinct epigenetic profiles have been associated with autism, and may mediate the link.[35] Whether or not genes are expressed depends on their regulation by other genes, which in turn depends on methylation (whether there is a methyl group attached to the DNA), imprinting (suppression of gene expression inherited from mother or father) and histones (the structures that chromosomes wind around), all of which may be influenced by the cellular environment, which in turn may be affected by cumulative exposure to toxins over the life course.[36] One review refers to evidence that three environmental exposures (polychlorinated biphenyls (found in paint), lead (found in petrol) and bisphenol A (found in plastic packaging)) can alter DNA methylation *in utero*.[37] Older parenthood means a person may have had more exposure to these substances, passing more epigenetic changes down the germline.[22] Whether longer exposure really results in permanent methylation changes or indeed whether methylation can be inherited across multiple generations in humans remains highly controversial.[38]

Pathway (iv) offers a credible socio-cultural explanation. As better parental education predicts later parenthood and is also probably correlated to autism awareness and the reporting of autism traits (pathway v), better parental education explains the link.[15] Education is a confounding factor; higher education predicts older parenthood and autism will be identified more often by those with higher education. Assuming parents with a better education are more likely to be aware of autism, analysis will reveal an artefactual correlation between the two.

A final possibility, perhaps the simplest, is that the observed association is due to inherited autistic traits. There is some evidence to suggest that, on average, people

Table 8.1 Plausibility check for older parenthood as a contributor to rise in autism

Increased in high-income countries?	Increased post-1990?	Substantial part of population?	Associated with neurodevelopmental outcomes, specifically autistic-type behaviours? (Is there plausible mechanism?)
Yes	Yes	Yes	Yes (Yes)

with autism are later in starting romantic relationships than allistic (non-autistic) people.[39] Studies suggest autistic adults are not only later in starting sexual relationships,[40] are less sexually experienced as adolescents and young adults,[41] have lower libido on average,[42] engage in inappropriate courtship behaviours and more often focus on inappropriate targets as potential mates.[43] Together, these studies suggest autistic people may face barriers in getting long-term sexual relationships off the ground and, if they eventually become parents, may be more likely to be older, passing on autistic traits in the second generation. The parent-with-traits pathway produces a putative looping or feedback mechanism (Figure 8.3). The social issues autistic people face in forming relationships feed back on to biological risk and, potentially, will increase the proportion of the population diagnosed with autism as the generations go by. The loop shown in Figure 8.3 cannot have contributed to the post-1990 rise in autism, however, as the timeframe is too short.

Could older parenthood *per se* plausibly explain any of the rise in autism? This is conceivable (Table 8.1) and may be due to any or all of the mechanisms shown in Figure 8.2, plus others. But the likelihood is that increasing parental age has had only a small impact on the rise in autism diagnosis. A study analysing nearly a million children born in New York between 1994 and 2001 found the proportion of mothers over 35 increased by around 15% and fathers over 35 increased by 12% in those seven years.[44] Autism prevalence in the cohort reportedly also increased, from 1 in 3,300 children born in 1994 to 1 in 233 children born in 2001. The risk of having a child with autism was nearly double for mothers aged 35 or older compared to those under 25 and nearly one and a half times greater for older fathers. Because they controlled for risk factors other than parental age, the researchers made the dubious calculation that parental age accounted for 2.7% of the rise in autism prevalence. Dubious, because the study was far from comprehensive in the 'risks' it was able to control for and made no attempt to account for changed understandings of autism, methods of identification, diagnostic infrastructures and cultural shifts. What the study did indicate is that it is plausible that a proportion of the rise in autism can be accounted for by older parenthood, but is likely to be dwarfed by the influence of other factors.

Air pollution

The time trend

Air pollution refers to concentrations of both dust and invisible gases. Most of what can be classified as 'pollutants' travels into the atmosphere from natural sources such as volcanic ashes, smoke from forest fires, pollen and hair; humans and animals are adapted to cope with these sources for example through mucous and cilia clearance.[45]

Human activities also release airborne particles, through the burning of forest and farmland, industrial pollution, domestic fires, energy production, agricultural emissions and especially through transport: planes, trains and automobiles.[45] Man-made pollutants in Africa are more likely to originate from domestic fires[46]; traffic, power generation and agricultural emissions contribute more in Europe, America and Asia.[47] Vehicles are estimated to be responsible for 30% of emissions of airborne particles and gases in European cities and up to 50% of emissions in the cities of lower-income countries, with older diesel vehicles the main culprits.[48] Gases, dust and ash emission particles may contain heavy metals, minerals, moulds, sulphur, carbon compounds and organic and chemicals, including benzene derivatives.

Particulate air pollution, airborne dust, is divided for analysis into smaller particles of fine particulate matter with an aerodynamic dry diameter of less than 2.5 micrometers (known as $PM_{2.5}$) and larger particles of particulate matter (PM_{10}). The bulk of research linking air pollution to neurodevelopmental outcomes has been carried out on $PM_{2.5}$.

An array of gases and particles, all with different toxicities, is lumped together as $PM_{2.5}$. Different emissions have different chemical compositions, so it is hard to detect a specific chemical signal for a possible neurodevelopment disruption mechanism. The diameter of the particle is not always the best determinant of how long it will remain airborne, nor of how the particle will interact with the respiratory system. In other words, a specific particle that may be damaging to human health may or may not be present in a generic measure of $PM_{2.5}$. Fibrous dusts, such as asbestos, can trigger distinct health problems but these are primarily related to the shape of the asbestos particles, not their size.[49] Furthermore, $PM_{2.5}$ levels are difficult to assess; they vary by time of day, indoors or outdoors, location, altitude, season, weather and local conditions.[50] The picture is further complicated in that people who may have experienced high exposure may not have frequent high exposure; prolonged low-level exposure may be more damaging than occasional high levels. Moreover, people of different ages have different sensitivities to pollution and human migration and travel render stable measurement of exposure even more challenging. The various methodological challenges of measuring air pollution have been summarised in several environmental papers.[51, 52]

Despite the difficulties in measurement, the time trend is well established. Levels of $PM_{2.5}$ in outdoor air have been increasing in low- and middle-income countries since the 1980s.[53] Emissions over Asia have increased notably, partly due to the existence of industrial plants and the use of diesel vehicles, especially in China and India. It is estimated that 87% of the global population lives in areas where the air quality exceeds the World Health Organization's (WHO) guidelines for annual mean ambient $PM_{2.5}$ (10 $\mu g/m^3$).[54]

However, in North America and Europe, levels of $PM_{2.5}$ have declined between 1990 and the present day.[55-57] US national data suggest levels have dropped consistently since 2000, although there is some evidence of a slight increase since 2016.[58] The trend towards better air quality in high-income countries is attributed to widespread implementation of air quality regulation and emission controls.[53]

Evidence of association

This cursory review gives a brief indication of the breadth of research on the putative association. Most epidemiological studies have focused on a child's pre-natal exposure or exposure during infancy – periods thought to be critical for the developing brain.[59] Much of the research on air pollution and child outcomes combines information from individual birth records or cohort data with measures of ambient air quality, usually from fixed outdoor monitors.[51] But because fixed monitors do not follow mothers around, this introduces a degree of measurement error. Studies that cover the mother's exposure to air pollution during pregnancy sometimes sub-divide the pregnancy by trimester to detect when the foetus might be more sensitive to air pollution but, to date, no systematic reviews have identified a clear pattern.[60] Pre-natal exposure is almost always assessed via maternal exposure to $PM_{2.5}$. This is problematic, as mothers vary in how efficient they are at removing inhaled particulate matter from their bodies before it is transferred to the foetus. Being a long-term smoker, for example, reduces the ability to remove particulate matter from the human system.[49] Studies cannot usually control for such varied ability.

Studies have produced mixed findings. A large Danish study of children born between 1989 and 2013 that included more than 15,000 children with an autism diagnosis and more than 68,000 controls matched by birth year found there was no association between maternal exposure to $PM_{2.5}$ during pregnancy and autism diagnosis in their offspring.[59] It did find that exposure to $PM_{2.5}$ in infancy increased the risk of autism diagnosis over and above the effect of parental age, smoking and pre-natal exposure to $PM_{2.5}$. Pollution was more strongly associated with autism among residents of urban neighbourhoods.[59]

Two smaller American studies (with approximately 250 cases of autism compared to roughly equal numbers of controls) from California[61] and Pennsylvania[62] assessed exposures to $PM_{2.5}$ pre- as well as post-natally. These studies both reported associations with autism risk during both developmental stages. The Californian study found exposure to heavy traffic pollution was significantly associated with a child's later research diagnosis.[63, 64] A study from China, on a similar scale, tested exposure in children's first three years of life and found positive correlations between severity of air pollution and autism.[65]

A big US study using satellite-based estimates of air quality, with a sample of more than two million eight-year-old children living in 15 US sites, found a positive correlation with air pollution exposure in pregnancy.[66] A smaller case-control study (more than 400 cases), based in Ohio, found a positive link between the risk of autism and post-natal exposure at high levels.[67] By contrast, another American study found absolutely no link between $PM_{2.5}$ exposure and autism severity,[68] and neither did a large Canadian study with a population-based sample of more than 100,000.[69] A pan-European study examining associations between exposure during gestation and autistic traits in four cohorts in the Netherlands, Spain, Italy and Sweden found no association.[70] A 2016 systematic review and meta-analysis found a significant increase in risk of autism when infants were exposed to higher levels of $PM_{2.5}$ but no overall effect for mothers' exposure during pregnancy.[71] However, only two studies met the inclusion criteria for the meta-analysis of infant exposure. A more recent systematic review,[60] using data from nine studies, estimated a small increased risk of autism was associated with pre-natal maternal exposure to $PM_{2.5}$ but it did not assess the post-natal effect of exposure. Overall, the evidence, although mixed, suggests there is a link.

My scoping search of the association between air pollution and neurodevelopmental outcomes revealed fewer studies about general neurodevelopment, perhaps because of the intense research focus on autism. The one systematic review I identified summarised links between neurodevelopmental outcomes, including cognitive functions, from 31 studies published between 2006 and 2015, covering associations with air pollution through the entire life course.[72] The vast majority of studies in the review came from high-income countries. Several studies included in this review found that pollution exposure *in utero* is associated with increased risk of neurodevelopmental delay; particulate exposure in childhood was associated with neurodevelopmental delays in younger children and with lower academic achievement and neurocognitive performance in older children.[72] In older adults, air pollution was associated with accelerated cognitive decline. The authors concluded there is not enough evidence to show definitive links, because the quality of the studies was patchy.

Possible mechanisms

The effects of poor air quality on health are far reaching but chiefly affect the lungs, breathing, the respiratory system and the heart and cardiovascular system.[45] Nevertheless, fine particulate air pollution can cross the blood–brain barrier and, in rodents, has been shown to induce structural and physiological damage.[73] The theorised biological pathways through which particulate air pollution induces neurodevelopmental disruption were helpfully summarised by Beate Ritz and colleagues.[59] Their non-exhaustive list includes gene–environment interaction, with elevated $PM_{2.5}$ exposure leading to *de novo* mutations,[74] epigenetic effects such as hypermethylation, leading to changes in oxidation and protein formation induced *in vitro* by exposure to $PM_{2.5}$.[75] Perhaps the chief theory is that particulate matter may have direct and indirect effects on brain tissue, through inflammation and oxidative stress.[76] One paper summarises a series of mechanistic investigations in which mice were exposed to high doses of ultrafine particles (a category of particles even smaller than $PM_{2.5}$).[73] These exposures induced a variety of inflammatory responses, including changes to mouse brain physiology and structure.

Several strong concerns have been raised concerning this type of work, particularly by the autistic community. First, can rodents really act as models for autism? In rodents, 'autistic' behaviours are modelled by observing the number and frequency of repetitive behaviours, aggression and social interaction. Autism is characterised by impairment in social communication, yet rodents have different social structures to humans and do not use language and gesture. Second, rodent experiments lack ecological validity, because the animals are kept in laboratory conditions rather than roaming free. Limited environmental stimulation in captive animals, such as in zoos, is known to induce repetitive behaviours.[77] Third, experimental conditions do not accurately replicate human experience; for example, in Allen and colleagues' study,[73] weaned mice were reportedly exposed to an average 96.4 µg/m³ of fine particles across the day, about four times the European Union legal limit for $PM_{2.5}$ (25 µg/m³ in 2019[78]). To give this above-daily-average exposure, extreme levels of fumigation must have been administered during the four-hour-long daily 'exposure' periods. The extremely high doses given to the developing mice are very unlike the everyday experience of most, if any, human infants.

Finally, the suffering of the animals involved is obscured by the scientific language used, which seems to distance us from the unpleasant reality and the impact on the animals. Being 'fumigated' for four hours at a time means the enforced breathing of highly polluted air every day. And after the study period, the mice are killed by decapitation. Despite the high pollution being described as a 'challenge' to the mice, the mice had no say in whether or not they were able to accept it.[79] Translating the behaviour of rodents and other animals across the species boundary to humans seems highly dubious. I personally find experiments that force mammals to repeatedly suffer high toxic exposures, then publish the unsurprising fact that they suffer brain damage, disturbing.

Could rising air pollution plausibly explain any of the rise in autism?

Unlikely (Table 8.2). $PM_{2.5}$ levels are dropping in high-income countries. If increased proximity to traffic fumes at local levels were partially responsible for the rise in autism due to more pregnant women and infants living near main roads, then there would also be evidence of increased premature deaths, known to be linked to air pollution. Instead, evidence suggests the numbers of premature deaths due to exposure to $PM_{2.5}$ have declined during 1990–2015 in Europe,[80] as $PM_{2.5}$ levels and other airborne pollutants have steadily dropped.[55–57]

In addition, the effect sizes reported by the systematic reviews are small. The latest review estimates a small increase in risk of having a baby diagnosed with autism for every 10 µg/m³ increase in $PM_{2.5}$ in the ambient pollution.[60] Given that the WHO's recommended guideline for *average* ambient $PM_{2.5}$ is 10 µg/m³,

Table 8.2 Plausibility check for PM$_{2.5}$ (small particulate matter)

Increased in high-income countries?	Increased post-1990?	Substantial part of population?	Associated with neurodevelopmental outcomes, specifically autistic-type behaviours? (Is there plausible mechanism?)
No	No	Yes	Yes (Yes)

this is a huge increase in pollution for a small increase in autism cases. Even in the biggest cities in high-income countries, an increase of 10 μg/m^3 is very substantial. In London in 2019, for example, average ambient PM$_{2.5}$ levels were approximately 10 μg/m^3 and around 12 μg/m^3 at busier roadsides. If levels of pollution did more or less double, so that the average level of PM$_{2.5}$ increased by 10 μg/m^3, this would be a horrendous increase in pollution but would result in only one more child in every 2,000 receiving an autism diagnosis, according to the estimate above.[60] In reality, London PM$_{2.5}$ levels have been going down by around 5 μg/m^3 every ten years.[78] This is not to say that particulate matter is not *per se* associated with autism; on balance, the evidence suggests it is, but it does not seem to be a plausible candidate to explain any of the observed rise in autism diagnoses in higher-income countries.

Pre-term birth

A baby is considered pre-term, or premature, if they are born before 37 weeks of gestation. Pre-term birth is further sub-divided according to gestational age. Extremely pre-term (before 28 weeks), very pre-term (28–32 weeks) and moderate pre-term or near-term birth (32–37 completed weeks of gestation) are the usual categories. Week by week, a foetus matures and if it doesn't fully develop in the womb, there is an amplified risk of multiple adverse and serious medical problems at birth. The shorter the gestation, the higher the risk of respiratory, heart and neurological problems, although this correlation diminishes as quality of neonatal care improves.[81] Even babies born near to term, at 37 or 38 weeks, who are not classed as pre-term, have higher risks of poor outcomes than those born at 40 weeks.[82] Premature birth can be spontaneous but often initiated because of medical issues during pregnancy, through a Caesarean or induced delivery. A ruptured membrane, and other pregnancy complications, is associated with increased risk of infection, which can prompt doctors to recommend early delivery.

Approximately one in ten children is born pre-term in the USA, the vast majority late pre-term. Late pre-term new-borns, born before but near the 37-week threshold, are the fastest-growing subset of neonates, accounting for approximately 74% of all pre-term births and about 8% of total births in 2010.[83] Late pre-term birth brings its own risks of neurological issues and heart and lung problems.[82] Increasingly, in some higher-income countries, a small proportion of babies are born pre-term for non-medical reasons, by elective pre-term

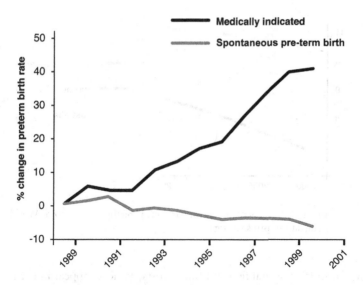

Figure 8.4 The time trend in medically induced /elective births in the USA. Percentage
change in rates relative to baseline rate in 1987 (index number, data from
Centers for Disease Control and Prevention).

Caesarean section, almost always carried out very near to the 37-week threshold.
US clinicians have reportedly become increasingly comfortable with births in late
pre-term gestations and many apparently recommend elective delivery or induced
labour well before 40 weeks of gestation, believing that neonates are as physio-
logically mature as full-term babies.[83] Figure 8.4 shows the trend toward more
medically initiated pre-term births.

Globally, around 10% of living babies are born pre-term.[82] In most countries
in Europe, in the USA and Australia, there was an overall drop in birth rates
between 1990 and 2020.[84–86] However, the estimated proportion of pre-term
births increased.[82,87] Figure 8.5 shows the increasing trend over time in pre-term
birth rates for these three regions.

In Europe, the perception that the proportion of pre-term births has uni-
formly increased has been questioned.[88] Most European countries have seen
increasing rates of pre-term birth since the mid-2000s but in some countries,
for example Finland and Sweden, pre-term birth rates have dropped.[88, 89] Thus,
continental trends mask considerable local and regional variation. In the USA,
the increase in late pre-term births has accounted for the birth of approximately
50,000 more infants since 1990.[90] But different districts within the USA have
distinct patterns, probably related to service delivery and other local cultural
factors.[90] Thresholds for acceptable length of gestation at delivery vary by region.
In Denmark, for example, a lower threshold of 22 weeks for extremely premature and viable replaced the 28-week cut-off in the mid-1990s. Furthermore,
in some countries babies who die soon after birth may be coded as stillborn, to

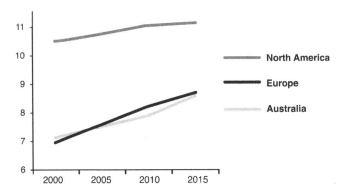

Figure 8.5 Time trend in percentage of pre-term births (data from World Health Organization: ptb.srhr.org).

minimise distress, hospital fees and burial costs, so never appear in the pre-term records.[91]

Despite the measurement, reporting, service provision and categorisation issues, it is still possible to see a clear overall trend by triangulating the data. Several sources, as well as the WHO data, establish an overall trend of more pre-term births since 1990.[82] Near-term birth has increased most in high-income countries and is generally accompanied by much milder difficulties than very pre-term birth; in these countries, near-term births account for the vast bulk of the rise in pre-term births. The proportion of medically initiated pre-term births is growing quickly, at least in the USA, partially due to greater demand for elective Caesarean section.[92, 93] Other drivers include fertility treatments such as *in vitro* fertilisation (IVF) and other assisted reproductive technologies, which produce more twins, triplets and other multiple births, which have a high (40–60%) chance of pre-term birth, compared with 5–10% for single deliveries.[94] Higher maternal age at childbirth is also associated with pre-term birth and may have contributed to the time trend.[88] Other predictors include higher maternal body mass index (particularly obesity) and diabetes, both of which are on the increase in many higher-income countries.[95–97] Interestingly, pre-term birth is more common for boys, with around 55% of all pre-term births occurring in boys.[98]

A picture emerges in which the majority of the 'new' pre-term births in higher-income countries use medical technologies such as induction or surgery, are medically initiated or elective and are near the boundary of pre-term, nearing full gestation. Very approximately, 1% more of all children born in high-income countries are now born pre-term than were in 1990 (Figure 8.5).

Evidence of association

Direct complications of pre-term birth are thought to account for one million deaths each year;[82] pre-term birth is the leading cause of child death globally.[82]

Conditions precipitated by premature birth include respiratory and cardiovascular disorders, and cognitive and neuro-disabilities.[99]

Most studies of neurodevelopmental, cognitive and behavioural outcomes have examined their association with very premature birth in extremely low-birth-weight babies. The survival of very pre-term infants has improved markedly over recent decades because of medical advances in neonatal care.[99] Human viability, currently approximately 23–24 weeks' gestation in most higher-income countries, is defined as gestational age at which the chance of survival is 50%[100] The length of gestation needed for a baby to be viable has dropped as medical technologies and services have improved over time.

Around half of infants born *very* pre-term in high-income countries survive but around half of the survivors have moderate to profound impairment at one to two years old.[101] The earlier the baby, the greater the risk. Of all children with cerebral palsy, around 45% will be pre-term.[81] Thus, although technology and medical interventions have pushed back the age at which babies are 'viable' survivors, so the very premature set of survivors is more likely to have cerebral palsy and other neurological conditions, although the extent is dependent on the quality of and access to local health care services.[102]

Most studies have concluded there is a strong association for pre-term children with a range of other neurodevelopmental, cognitive and behavioural outcomes as they grow up. An Australian study of approximately 500 cases and controls, comparing outcomes of full-term and very pre-term children, found the latter had worse outcomes on a range of behavioural and cognitive measures at school age.[103] The very pre-term group seem particularly vulnerable to difficulties related to inattention and hyperactivity and may have emotional troubles at school age that affect academic performance,[104] and the risk of ID is high.[105] One US study of around 4,500 infants born between 22 and 25 weeks' gestation found 73% had either died or had impairment before they were two years old.[105] The ethics of keeping very pre-term children, of so-called 'borderline viability', alive through neonatal intervention is therefore debated in medical journals in terms of risk to the children, their quality of life, and their families and the cost to wider society.[106]

However, the vast majority of pre-term births occur near term, and this group accounts for most of the increasing pre-term birth rate in higher-income countries.[83] Could this potentially be a driver for more autism cases? In some countries, including France, the proportion of late pre-term infants with serious problems has decreased as time has passed, probably due to better care.[107] Nevertheless, in mainstream school settings, children in the late pre-term group still have lower scores, on average, than full-term children on a range of measures.[108–110] A systematic review concluded a range of neurodevelopmental outcomes was 'better' in children with full-term gestation compared to those born before full term, even if the difference in gestation was only a couple of weeks.[111] Three of the studies in this review found a significant association between ADHD and late pre-term birth. Intriguingly, in two, the effect was only seen when delivery was medically induced.[111]

Autism has been repeatedly linked to very pre-term birth and to very low birth weight. One meta-analysis that included 18 studies from Japan, South Korea,

Belgium and Saudi Arabia, examined the prevalence of autism in more than 3,000 pre-term infants (mostly very pre-term) and concluded that there is a higher prevalence of autism in pre-term children than in full-term children.[112] Autism has also been associated with low birth weight, a proxy measure for prematurity, in many studies.[17, 113-117] Overall, though there is strong evidence that autism is associated with very pre-term birth, for children born nearer to term, who account for the bulk of extra pre-term births, there is less evidence, although one review of reviews cited Ceasarian section as an established risk factor for autism.[125]

Possible mechanisms

A common hypothesis of how brain development may be disrupted in pre-term children appears to implicate hypoxia, a lack of oxygen reaching the brain, induced by immature lung development. The lack of oxygen after birth can lead to brain damage, which quickly causes injury to vulnerable neurons and the physiology of the new-born brain.[118] The brain regions involved in cognitive functioning, the hippocampus and cortex, are often damaged by hypoxia at or after birth.[119] Early umbilical cord clamping, an under-researched risk factor put forward by a midwife in our original study, seems a plausible trigger.[14] Unfortunately, data on early cord clamping seem hard to obtain.

Could the rise in pre-term births plausibly explain any of the rise in autism?

Possibly. The evidence that autism is associated with later pre-term births has been hard to find (Table 8.3). The increase in pre-term births since 1990 in high-income countries is largely driven by babies born at or near term. The one meta-analysis I found specifically on the association between autism and pre-term birth had a median gestation of 28 weeks, so the majority of babies included were not in the late pre-term or near-term categories.[112] Digging deeper into the studies in the review reveals a Belgian study that found 40% of infants had autism at two years old.[120] Closer inspection shows *all* the pre-term children in the Belgian study were born very pre-term, at fewer than 27 weeks' gestation. Another cohort study from Finland found no increased risk of autism with birth beyond 32 weeks' gestation.[121] The conclusion of the review, that 900,000 children have autism accounted for by recent rises in pre-term births, is probably a gross over-estimate, because it is based on the premise that pre-term birth is *per se* a risk factor for autism, without reference to the more serious risk conferred by being born very pre-term rather than nearer term.[122]

Late pre-term births are, however, associated with cognitive delay and worse academic outcomes than in full-term children. This suggests there may be milder neurodevelopmental complications for this group. As the rise in autism is primarily due to an increase in higher-functioning children, there may be an interaction between rising late-pre term births and the trend to diagnose milder impairment.[123]

Table 8.3 Plausibility check for late pre-term birth as a risk factor

Increased in high-income countries?	Increased post-1990?	Substantial part of population?	Associated with neurodevelopmental outcomes, specifically autistic-type behaviours? (Is there plausible mechanism?)
Yes	Yes	Yes	Maybe (Yes)

An aside: The headless mother

It is striking that pregnant women rarely appear in the pregnancy risk literature as actual people; they more often become the 'maternal environment'. To maximise their chance of having a normal, thriving child, it is the maternal environment's responsibility to take medical advice, regulate its diet and alcohol intake, avoid smoking and other potentially dangerous exposures, and endorse and uphold medical and community regulation of its body.

The risk literature contributes to the apparent community ownership of pregnant bodies. Writing of the uterus as public theatre, Rebecca Kukla discusses how the literature on the effect of environmental contaminants, such as $PM_{2.5}$, during pregnancy qualifies pregnant bodies as public spaces.[124] Bearing a healthy child is 'for the public good', whereas pregnant women's own outcomes are rarely considered. The emphasis on women controlling their bodies to protect the unborn child means that threats to the woman herself, whether through poverty, domestic violence or health risks, are obscured, she argues. The emphasis on the unborn child underlines its importance; the importance of the woman is as the vessel to carry it. Thus, the dominant discourse of risk in the epidemiological literature is concerned with risk to the foetal health and it throws its weight behind public health interventions designed to change women's behaviour and protect the unborn child.

This discourse of risk props up gendered power relations: the subordination of women, the public ownership of the pregnant body, heightened requirements for female self-surveillance during pregnancy, female culpability and dehumanising images of the pregnant torso cut off at the neck. Women's adherence, or lack of adherence, to obligatory behaviour – what they eat, what they expose themselves to – becomes the source of risk, at the expense of more overtly political concerns around population-level determinants of foetal health, including economic, social and nutritional inequalities.

Other risks

My brief review of three of the lay epidemiologists' candidate risk factors suggests that some may plausibly be implicated in the rise of autism diagnosis. But many other candidate social and environmental risk factors, stemming from medical technologies, built environments and environmental contaminants, have been studied. A recent review of reviews by Amirhossein Modabbernia and colleagues which, by its own admission, uses a design that provided only 'a wide view of the evidence landscape in epidemiology', is a useful pointer.[125] Hitherto under-researched risk factors such as early cord clamping and low-level radiation (both put forward by two of the lay epidemiologists), that may be salient, are absent in the review of reviews due to lack of attention.

Modabbernia's review concluded there is compelling evidence that greater paternal age, birth complications (including hypoxia and Caesarean section) and vitamin D deficiency are associated with autism, although one paper linking autism and vitamin D was recently retracted.[125] The review noted that links between environmental lead, mercury and autism were not proven but the evidence warranted further investigation (mercury amalgam dental fillings were implicated by one lay epidemiologist). Some drugs administered during pregnancy, for example the anti-epilepsy drug sodium valproate, are strongly associated with autism in offspring. The effects of valproate have been known since the 1970s but this information wasn't made widely available until years later, prompting calls in the UK for government apology.

The review found studies of diet were generally low-quality, offering little evidence of links to autism. However, a growing amount of research suggests that changes in the gastro-intestinal tract may affect the brain, through the two-way communication known as the gut–brain axis; for example, people suffering from inflammatory bowel disease are twice as likely to develop dementia.[126] The review also points to exposure to endocrine-disrupting chemicals, giving the example of bromide flame retardants (which increase free testosterone) in tandem with increased risk of autism.[125] Both gut–brain and hormone-disrupting exposures are areas in which further investigation is needed.

These conclusions are similar to those of Craig Newschaffer and colleagues, who wrote several major reviews about the environmental aetiology of autism during the 1990s and 2000s.[127, 128] In particular, Newschaffer's team identified maternal infections during pregnancy as a risk factor. Another recent review finds evidence for bacterial infection and flu during pregnancy as elevating the risk of autism.[129] No doubt Covid-19 infection during pregnancy will be a future site of research into the risk of autism and broader neuro-disability.

Real risks and artefacts

Reviews and meta-analyses have shown that pre-term birth, older parents, infection during pregnancy and birth complications are associated with higher incidence of autism in offspring.[125] Caesarean section, which has led to more pre-term births and is itself a facet of medicalisation, has been directly linked to autism.[125]

Caution must be exercised when interpreting results. In any association study, it is not really possible to sort out what causes what. One problem is confounding; take the example of air pollution (as the exposure) and its association with autism (as the outcome). People who live in more polluted places tend to be more socially and economically disadvantaged than those who live in less

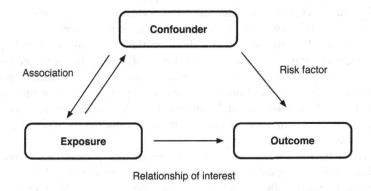

Figure 8.6 Confounding in epidemiology.

polluted settings but this difference is itself associated with many other lifestyle differences: diet, smoking, depression, younger parenthood and obesity, to name a few. None of these differences is caused by the pollution and it could be that one or more of them is explanatory of difference in rates of autism diagnosis. To take the example further, let's say obesity is linked to a greater likelihood of birth complications that increase the chances of hypoxia, thus increasing the chance of autism in the offspring. Obesity is a confounder; it is linked both to the exposure (air pollution) and, via the risk factor (hypoxia), to autism (the outcome). This hypothetical example illustrates how associations that are spurious, or artefacts of other associations, are sometimes reported (Figure 8.6).

Epidemiologists try to control for many such factors but it is not always clear how effective their designs are. Most study designs don't control for many unobserved or unmeasured factors. Confounding means there may be a mediator which is a stronger determinant, causing spurious or artefactual associations. That is why the mantra of the epidemiologist is 'correlation is not causality'.

Another problem is 'collinearity', which means the predictors of risk are correlated. This can inflate the estimation of risk. The three risk factors I have examined (older parents, pre-term birth and air pollution), are correlated. Babies with older parents are more likely to have low birth weight and be born prematurely. Exposure to air pollution in pregnancy is a predictor for low birth weight and pre-term birth. It also predicts that the child will be exposed to air pollution after birth. All three risk factors have been associated with hypoxia, which itself is a well-researched risk factor for autism that could mediate the effects.[125]

A third issue is that measurements of different categories of risk vary and thresholds for defining categories may change over time; as we saw earlier, what counts as 'pre-term' varies among countries and over time. Missing data is yet another issue, especially in longitudinal association studies, such as births of stillborn children or those who die soon after birth being poorly recorded or missing in some countries, for cultural or pragmatic reasons.[91] In Europe, and in anglophone countries, the drop-out rate of participants in longitudinal studies that link earlier exposures to later outcomes is clearly linked to socio-economic disadvantage, which itself maybe linked to the outcome of interest.[130]

The Covid-19 crisis has shone a light on the variations in recording and reporting health statistics among nations. Levels of missing data are often highest in low-income countries, as they have fewer resources to allow them to participate in research studies and undertake less testing or surveying of their population. Covid-19 has also raised the question of whether the death figures may be subject to 'massaging' or interference in more authoritative states anxious to protect their international reputation.

Layered over these inherent uncertainties are the politics of research and funding. Epidemiologists' attention to a particular risk factor and/or outcome seems to be directed by the *zeitgeist*.[91] For example, research attention to air pollution has consistently increasingly been directed at $PM_{2.5}$, an arbitrary diameter; a bibliometric review of $PM_{2.5}$ research found research on it grew exponentially between 1997 and 2016.[131] But it may be that particle shape, or the precise composition of the chemicals that make up the particulate mix, is more relevant to health outcomes. $PM_{2.5}$ increasingly became a focus of research at the expense of different substrates within $PM_{2.5}$, as well as other forms of air pollution. This bibliographic study[131] is reminiscent of the work of Jennifer Singh and colleagues, which demonstrated a huge increase in research funding about autism over the same time period.[132] Funding for autism research from the US National Institutes of Health increased five-fold between 1997 and 2006, from $22 million to $108 million, and continues to climb.[132]

Singh studies how entities such as autism become salient and maintain themselves as sites of knowledge production, seeding centres and funding, journals and research staff to become important areas of investigation. Knowledge about autism and activity around it can loop back into rising referrals and rising diagnosis. Conducting the literature review for this chapter, I recognised clusters of research groups in different parts of the world repeatedly publishing on one topic: air pollution in California, rodent models in China, and so on. As influential research groups gain and lose momentum and funding, they determine what is studied and therefore in what directions and down which channels our knowledge flows. Knowledge seems fluid and flowing, like a stream breaking off in different directions from the main channel of a river, shifting course over geological time. Some areas will begin to have more research interest than others and, as they do, funding will enrich them, like rain does a river. The reality shifts depending from which stream of knowledge it originates, and why, perhaps, Ian Hacking described the word 'real' as one of the great 'ideological' words.[133] This, and the more concrete evaluation of uncertainties inherent in epidemiology, suggests that measurement of risk is itself subject to artefactual shifts. This is not to say that risks do not exist or should not be quantified, rather that their quantification is influenced by the circumstances of their measurement.

In the Introduction, I identified a debate between those who think there are 'real' components to the rise in autism diagnoses and those who do not.

Artefactual changes involve shifting boundaries, creating either a bigger category or one applied to more types of people. A 'real' effect, I argued, means that there have been increased risk factors that seed the more real neurodevelopmental differences diagnosed as autism. Association studies seeking to identify such risk factors, using autism as an outcome against which to quantify risk of exposures, can themselves be victims of artefactual measurement, category and interpretative errors. Alternatively, new definitions of what counts as autism are equally 'real' and the fact that that there are additional types of people who can qualify as having autism is 'real' too. In these ways, the boundaries between what is real and what is artefact break down on closer inspection.

References

1. Craig, F. *et al.* A Review of Executive Function Deficits in Autism Spectrum Disorder and Attention-deficit/Hyperactivity Disorder. *Neuropsychiatr. Dis. Treat.* **12**, 1191–1202 (2016).
2. Cheung, C. H. M. *et al.* Aetiology for the Covariation Between Combined Type ADHD and Reading Difficulties in a Family Study: The Role of IQ. *J. Child Psychol. Psychiatry* **53**, 864–873 (2012).
3. van der Meer, J. M. J. *et al.* Are Autism Spectrum Disorder and Attention-deficit/Hyperactivity Disorder Different Manifestations of one Overarching Disorder? Cognitive and Symptom Evidence from a Clinical and Population-based Sample. *J. Am. Acad. Child Adolesc. Psychiatry* **51**, 1160–1172. e3 (2012).
4. Jeste, S. S. & Tuchman, R. Autism Spectrum Disorder and Epilepsy: Two Sides of the Same Coin? *J. Child Neurol.* **30**, 1963–1971 (2015).
5. Reiersen, A. M. & Todd, R. D. Co-occurrence of ADHD and Autism Spectrum Disorders: Phenomenology and Treatment. *Expert Rev. Neurother.* **8**, 657–669 (2008).
6. Einfeld, S. L., Ellis, L. A. & Emerson, E. Comorbidity of Intellectual Disability and Mental Disorder in Children and Adolescents: A Systematic Review. *J. Intellect. Dev. Disabil.* **36**, 137–143 (2011).
7. Hallett, V., Ronald, A. & Happe, F. Investigating the Association Between Autistic-like and Internalizing Traits in a Community-based Twin Sample. *J. Am. Acad. Child Adolesc. Psychiatry* **48**, 618–627 (2009).
8. Kerns, C. M. & Kendall, P. C. The Presentation and Classification of Anxiety in Autism Spectrum Disorder. *Clin. Psychol. Sci. Pract.* **19**, 323–347 (2012).
9. Muris, P., Steerneman, P., Merckelbach, H., Holdrinet, I. & Meesters, C. Comorbid Anxiety Symptoms in Children with Pervasive Developmental Disorders. *J. Anxiety Disord.* **12**, 387–393 (1998).
10. Grzadzinski, R. *et al.* Examining Autistic Traits in Children with ADHD: Does the Autism Spectrum Extend to ADHD? *J. Autism Dev. Disord.* **41**, 1178–1191 (2011).
11. Loomes, R., Hull, L. & Mandy, W. P. L. What is the Male-to-Female Ratio in Autism Spectrum Disorder? A Systematic Review and Meta-Analysis. *J. Am. Acad. Child Adolesc. Psychiatry* **56**, 466–474 (2017).
12. Symes, W. & Humphrey, N. Peer-group Indicators of Social Inclusion Among Pupils with Autistic Spectrum Disorders (ASD) in Mainstream Secondary Schools: A Comparative Study. *Sch. Psychol. Int.* **31**, 478–494 (2010). doi:10.1177/0143034310382496.

13. Daniels, J. L. *et al.* Parental Psychiatric Disorders Associated with Autism Spectrum Disorders in the Offspring. *Pediatrics* **121**, e1357–e1362 (2008).

14. Russell, G., Kelly, S. & Golding, J. A Qualitative Analysis of Lay Beliefs About the Aetiology and Prevalence of Autistic Spectrum Disorders. *Child Care Health Dev.* **36**, 431–436 (2010). doi:10.1111/j.1365-2214.2009.00994.x.

15. Bui, Q. & Miller, C. C. The Age That Women Have Babies: How a Gap Divides America. *The New York Times* (4 August 2018).

16. Barclay, K. & Myrskylä, M. Advanced Maternal Age and Offspring Outcomes: Reproductive Aging and Counterbalancing Period Trends. *Popul. Dev. Rev.* **42**, 69–94 (2016).

17. Russell, G., Steer, C. & Golding, J. Social and Demographic Factors That Influence the Diagnosis of Autistic Spectrum Disorders. *Soc. Psychiatry Psychiatr. Epidemiol.* **46**, 1283–1293 (2011).

18. Parner, E. T. *et al.* Parental Age and Autism Spectrum Disorders. *Ann. Epidemiol.* **22**, 143–150 (2012).

19. Grice, D. *et al.* Parental Age and Differential Risk For ASD, ADHD, OCD and Tic Disorders: Data From a Large National Cohort. *Eur. Neuropsychopharmacol.* **27**, S492 (2017).

20. King, M. D., Fountain, C., Dakhlallah, D. & Bearman, P. S. Estimated Autism Risk and Older Reproductive Age. *Am. J. Public Health* **99**, 1673–1679 (2009).

21. Idring, S. *et al.* Parental Age and the Risk of Autism Spectrum Disorders: Findings from a Swedish Population-based Cohort. *Int. J. Epidemiol.* **43**, 107–115 (2014).

22. Hultman, C. M., Sandin, S., Levine, S. Z., Lichtenstein, P. & Reichenberg, A. Advancing Paternal Age and Risk of Autism: New Evidence from a Population-based Study and a Meta-analysis of Epidemiological Studies. *Mol. Psychiatry* **16**, 1203–1212 (2011).

23. Sandin, S. *et al.* Advancing Maternal Age is Associated with Increasing Risk for Autism: A Review and Meta-analysis. *J. Am. Acad. Child Adolesc. Psychiatry* **51**, 477–486.e1 (2012).

24. Wu, S. *et al.* Advanced Parental Age and Autism Risk in Children: A Systematic Review and Meta-analysis. *Acta Psychiatr. Scand.* **135**, 29–41 (2017).

25. Saha, S. *et al.* Advanced Paternal Age is Associated with Impaired Neurocognitive Outcomes during Infancy and Childhood. *PLoS Med.* **6**, e1000040 (2009).

26. Morris, J. K., Mutton, D. E. & Alberman, E. Revised Estimates of the Maternal Age Specific Live Birth Prevalence of Down's Syndrome. *J. Med. Screen.* (2016) doi:10.1136/jms.9.1.2.

27. Johnson, K. J. *et al.* Parental Age and Risk of Childhood Cancer: A Pooled Analysis. *Epidemiol. Camb. Mass.* **20**, 475–483 (2009).

28. Sutcliffe, A. G., Barnes, J., Belsky, J., Gardiner, J. & Melhuish, E. The Health and Development of Children Born to Older Mothers in the United Kingdom: Observational Study Using Longitudinal Cohort Data. *BMJ* **345** (2012).

29. Sebat, J. *et al.* Strong Association of De Novo Copy Number Mutations with Autism. *Science* **316**, 445–449 (2007).

30. Marshall, C. R. *et al.* Structural Variation of Chromosomes in Autism Spectrum Disorder. *Am. J. Hum. Genet.* **82**, 477–488 (2008).

31. Deweerdt, S. Age and Autism – The Link Between Parental Age and Autism, Explained. www.spectrumnews.org/news/link-parental-age-autism-explained/.

32. Jolly, M., Sebire, N., Harris, J., Robinson, S. & Regan, L. The Risks Associated with Pregnancy in Women Aged 35 Years or Older. *Hum. Reprod. Oxf. Engl.* **15**, 2433–2437 (2000).

33. Pascal, A. *et al.* Neurodevelopmental Outcome in Very Preterm and Very-low-birthweight Infants Born over the Past Decade: A Meta-analytic Review. *Dev. Med. Child Neurol.* **60**, 342–355 (2018).

34. Goisis, A., Schneider, D. C. & Myrskylä, M. Secular Changes in the Association Between Advanced Maternal Age and the Risk of Low Birth Weight: A Cross-cohort Comparison in the UK. *Popul. Stud.* **72**, 381–397 (2018).

35. Schanen, N. C. Epigenetics of Autism Spectrum Disorders. *Hum. Mol. Genet.* **15**, R138–R150 (2006).

36. Yauk, C. et al. Germ-line Mutations, DNA Damage, and Global Hypermethylation in Mice Exposed to Particulate Air Pollution in an Urban/Industrial Location. *Proc. Natl Acad. Sci. USA* **105**, 605–610 (2008).

37. Keil, K. P. & Lein, P. J. DNA Methylation: A Mechanism Linking Environmental Chemical Exposures to Risk of Autism Spectrum Disorders? *Environ. Epigenetics* **2** (2016) dvv012.

38. Horsthemke, B. A Critical View on Transgenerational Epigenetic Inheritance in Humans. *Nat. Commun.* **9**, 1–4 (2018).

39. Barnett, J. P. & Maticka-Tyndale, E. Qualitative Exploration of Sexual Experiences Among Adults on the Autism Spectrum: Implications for Sex Education. *Perspect. Sex. Reprod. Health* **47**, 171–179 (2015).

40. Sala, G., Hooley, M. & Stokes, M. A. Romantic Intimacy in Autism: A Qualitative Analysis. *J. Autism Dev. Disord.* (2020) doi:10.1007/s10803-020-04377-8.

41. Dewinter, J., Vermeiren, R., Vanwesenbeeck, I. & Van Nieuwenhuizen, Ch. Adolescent Boys with Autism Spectrum Disorder Growing Up: Follow-up of Self-reported Sexual Experience. *Eur. Child Adolesc. Psychiatry* **25**, 969–978 (2016).

42. Bejerot, S. & Eriksson, J. M. Sexuality and Gender Role in Autism Spectrum Disorder: A Case Control Study. *PLoS One* **9** (2014) e87961.

43. Stokes, M., Newton, N. & Kaur, A. Stalking, and Social and Romantic Functioning Among Adolescents and Adults with Autism Spectrum Disorder. *J. Autism Dev. Disord.* **37**, 1969–1986 (2007).

44. Quinlan, C. A., McVeigh, K. H., Driver, C. R., Govind, P. & Karpati, A. Parental Age and Autism Spectrum Disorders Among New York City Children 0–36 Months of Age. *Matern. Child Health J.* **19**, 1783–1790 (2015).

45. Vallero, D. *Fundamentals of Air Pollution, 4th Edition* (Academic Press, 2007).

46. Butt, E. W. *et al.* The Impact of Residential Combustion Emissions on Atmospheric Aerosol, Human Health, and Climate. *Atmospheric Chem. Phys.* **16**, 873–905 (2016).

47. Lelieveld, J., Evans, J. S., Fnais, M., Giannadaki, D. & Pozzer, A. The Contribution of Outdoor Air Pollution Sources to Premature Mortality on a Global Scale. *Nature* **525**, 367–371 (2015).

48. WHO. Air Pollution. WHO. www.who.int/health-topics/air-pollution#tab=tab_1

49. WHO. Dust, Hazard Prevention and Control in the Work Environment: Airborne Dust. www.who.int/occupational_health/publications/airdust/en/

50. Leung, D. Y. C. Outdoor–indoor Air Pollution in Urban Environment: Challenges and Opportunity. *Front. Environ. Sci.* **2** (2015).

51. Woodruff, T. J. *et al.* Methodological Issues in Studies of Air Pollution and Reproductive Health. *Environ. Res.* **109**, 311–320 (2009).

52. Ren, C. & Tong, S. Health Effects of Ambient Air Pollution – Recent Research Development and Contemporary Methodological Challenges. *Environ. Health* **7**(56), (2008).

53. Butt, E. W. *et al*. Global and Regional Trends in Particulate Air Pollution and Attributable Health Burden over the Past 50 Years. *Environ. Res. Lett.* **12**, 104017 (2017).

54. Apte, J. S., Marshall, J. D., Cohen, A. J. & Brauer, M. Addressing Global Mortality from Ambient $PM_{2.5}$. *Environ. Sci. Technol.* **49**, 8057–8066 (2015).

55. Leibensperger, E. M. *et al*. Climatic Effects of 1950–2050 Changes in US Anthropogenic Aerosols – Part 1: Aerosol Trends and Radiative Forcing. *Atmospheric Chem. Phys.* **12**, 3349–3362 (2012).

56. Tørseth, K. *et al*. Introduction to the European Monitoring and Evaluation Programme (EMEP) and Observed Atmospheric Composition Change. *Atmospheric Chem. Phys.* **12**, 5447–5481 (2012).

57. Turnock, S. T. *et al*. Modelled and Observed Changes in Aerosols and Surface Solar Radiation over Europe Between 1960 and 2009. *Atmospheric Chem. Phys.* **15**, 9477–9500 (2015).

58. Clay, K. & Muller, N. Z. *Recent Increases in Air Pollution: Evidence and Implications for Mortality*. www.nber.org/papers/w26381 doi:10.3386/w26381 (2019).

59. Ritz, B. *et al*. Air Pollution and Autism in Denmark. *Environ. Epidemiol. Phila. Pa* **2** (2018) e028.

60. Chun, H., Leung, C., Wen, S. W., McDonald, J. & Shin, H. H. Maternal Exposure to Air Pollution and Risk of Autism in Children: A Systematic Review and Meta-analysis. *Environ. Pollut.* **256**, 113307 (2020).

61. Volk, H. E., Lurmann, F., Penfold, B., Hertz-Picciotto, I. & McConnell, R. Traffic Related Air Pollution, Particulate Matter, and Autism. *JAMA Psychiatry* **70**, 71–77 (2013).

62. Talbott, E. O. *et al*. Fine Particulate Matter and the Risk of Autism Spectrum Disorder. *Environ. Res.* **140**, 414–420 (2015).

63. Volk, H. E., Hertz-Picciotto, I., Delwiche, L., Lurmann, F. & McConnell, R. Residential Proximity to Freeways and Autism in the CHARGE Study. *Environ. Health Perspect.* **119**, 873–877 (2011).

64. Becerra, T. A., Wilhelm, M., Olsen, J., Cockburn, M. & Ritz, B. Ambient Air Pollution and Autism in Los Angeles County, California. *Environ. Health Perspect.* **121**, 380–386 (2013).

65. Geng, R., Fang, S. & Li, G. The Association Between Particulate Matter 2.5 Exposure and Children with Autism Spectrum Disorder. *Int. J. Dev. Neurosci. Off. J. Int. Soc. Dev. Neurosci.* **75**, 59–63 (2019).

66. Al-Hamdan, A. Z., Preetha, P. P., Albashaireh, R. N., Al-Hamdan, M. Z. & Crosson, W. L. Investigating the Effects of Environmental Factors on Autism Spectrum Disorder in the USA Using Remotely Sensed Data. *Environ. Sci. Pollut. Res. Int.* **25**, 7924–7936 (2018).

67. Kaufman, J. A. *et al*. Ambient Ozone and Fine Particulate Matter Exposures and Autism Spectrum Disorder in Metropolitan Cincinnati, Ohio. *Environ. Res.* **171**, 218–227 (2019).

68. Kerin, T. *et al*. Association Between Air Pollution Exposure, Cognitive and Adaptive Function, and ASD Severity Among Children with Autism Spectrum Disorder. *J. Autism Dev. Disord.* **48**, 137–150 (2018).

69. Pagalan, L. *et al*. Association of Prenatal Exposure to Air Pollution With Autism Spectrum Disorder. *JAMA Pediatr.* **173**, 86–92 (2019).

70. Guxens M. *et al*. Air Pollution Exposure during Pregnancy and Childhood Autistic Traits in Four European Population-Based Cohort Studies: The ESCAPE Project. *Environ. Health Perspect.* **124**, 133–140 (2016).

71. Flores-Pajot, M.-C., Ofner, M., Do, M. T., Lavigne, E. & Villeneuve, P. J. Childhood Autism Spectrum Disorders and Exposure to Nitrogen Dioxide, and Particulate Matter Air Pollution: A Review and Meta-analysis. *Environ. Res.* **151**, 763–776 (2016).

72. Clifford, A., Lang, L., Chen, R., Anstey, K. J. & Seaton, A. Exposure to Air Pollution and Cognitive Functioning Across the Life Course – A Systematic Literature Review. *Environ. Res.* **147**, 383–398 (2016).

73. Allen, J. L. *et al.* Developmental Neurotoxicity of Inhaled Ambient Ultrafine Particle Air Pollution: Parallels with Neuropathological and Behavioral Features of Autism and other Neurodevelopmental Disorders. *NeuroToxicology* **59**, 140–154 (2017).

74. Kim, D. *et al.* The Joint Effect of Air Pollution Exposure and Copy Number Variation on Risk for Autism. *Autism Res. Off. J. Int. Soc. Autism Res.* **10**, 1470–1480 (2017).

75. Wei, H. *et al.* Redox/methylation Mediated Abnormal DNA Methylation as Regulators of Ambient Fine Particulate Matter-induced Neurodevelopment Related Impairment In Human Neuronal Cells. *Sci. Rep.* **6**, 33402 (2016).

76. Block, M. L. & Calderón-Garcidueñas, L. Air Pollution: Mechanisms of Neuroinflammation and CNS Disease. *Trends Neurosci.* **32**, 506–516 (2009).

77. Mason, G. Stereotypic Behaviour in Captive Animals: Fundamentals and Implications for Welfare and Beyond. In *Stereotypic Animal Behaviour: Fundamentals and Applications to Welfare* (eds. Mason, G. & Rushen, J.) 325–356 (CABI, 2006). doi:10.1079/9780851990040.0325.

78. Mayor of London. *PM$_{2.5}$ in London: Roadmap to Meeting World Health Organization Guidelines by 2030* (Greater London Authority, 2019).

79. Allen, J. L. *et al.* Developmental Exposure to Concentrated Ambient Particles and Preference for Immediate Reward in Mice. *Environ. Health Perspect.* **121**, 32–38 (2013).

80. Ciarelli, G. *et al.* Long-term Health Impact Assessment of Total PM$_{2.5}$ in Europe During the 1990–2015 Period. Atmospheric Environ. X **3**, 100032 (2019).

81. Allen, M. C. Neurodevelopmental Outcomes of Preterm Infants. *Curr. Opin. Neurol.* **21**, 123–128 (2008).

82. Blencowe, H. *et al.* Born Too Soon: The Global Epidemiology of 15 Million Preterm Births. *Reprod. Health* **10**, S2 (2013) (Suppl 1): S2.

83. Loftin, R. W. *et al.* Late Preterm Birth. *Rev. Obstet. Gynecol.* **3**, 10–19 (2010).

84. Macrotrends. U.K. Birth Rate 1950–2020. www.macrotrends.net/countries/GBR/united-kingdom/birth-rate.

85. Macrotrends. Australia Birth Rate 1950–2020. www.macrotrends.net/countries/AUS/australia/birth-rate.

86. Macrotrends. U.S. Birth Rate 1950–2020. www.macrotrends.net/countries/USA/united-states/birth-rate.

87. Chawanpaiboon, S. *et al.* Global, Regional, and National Estimates of Levels of Preterm Birth in 2014: A Systematic Review and Modelling Analysis. *Lancet Glob. Health* 7, e37–e46 (2019).

88. Zeitlin, J. *et al.* Preterm Birth Time Trends in Europe: A Study of 19 Countries. *BJOG Int. J. Obstet. Gynaecol.* **120**, 1356–1365 (2013).

89. Richards, J. L. *et al.* Temporal Trends in Late Preterm and Early Term Birth Rates in 6 High-Income Countries in North America and Europe and Association With Clinician-Initiated Obstetric Interventions. *JAMA* **316**, 410–419 (2016).

90. Martin, J. A., Kirmeyer, S., Osterman, M. & Shepherd, R. A. Born a Bit Too Early: Recent Trends in Late Preterm Births. *NCHS Data Brief* 1–8 (2009).

91. Lumley, J. Defining the Problem: The Epidemiology of Preterm Birth. *BJOG Int. J. Obstet. Gynaecol.* **110**, 3–7 (2003).

92. VanderWeele, T. J., Lantos, J. D. & Lauderdale, D. S. Rising Preterm Birth Rates, 1989–2004: Changing Demographics or Changing Obstetric Practice? *Soc. Sci. Med.* **74**, 196–201 (2012).

93. Zhang, X. & Kramer, M. S. The Rise in Singleton Preterm Births in the USA: The Impact of Labour Induction. *BJOG Int. J. Obstet. Gynaecol.* **119**, 1309–1315 (2012).

94. Ooki, S. The Effect of an Increase in the Rate of Multiple Births on Low-birth-weight and Preterm Deliveries during 1975–2008. *J. Epidemiol.* **20**, 480–488 (2010).

95. Keirse, M. J. N. C., Hanssens, M. & Devlieger, H. Trends in Preterm Births in Flanders, Belgium, from 1991 to 2002. *Paediatr. Perinat. Epidemiol.* **23**, 522–532 (2009).

96. Tracy, S. K., Tracy, M. B., Dean, J., Laws, P. & Sullivan, E. Spontaneous Preterm Birth of Liveborn Infants in Women at Low Risk in Australia over 10 Years: A Population-based Study. *BJOG Int. J. Obstet. Gynaecol.* **114**, 731–735 (2007).

97. Steer, P. The Epidemiology of Preterm Labour. *BJOG Int. J. Obstet. Gynaecol.* **112**, 1–3 (2005).

98. Zeitlin, J. *et al.* Fetal Sex and Preterm Birth: Are Males at Greater Risk? *Hum. Reprod. Oxf. Engl.* **17**, 2762–2768 (2002).

99. Saigal, S. & Doyle, L. W. An Overview of Mortality and Sequelae of Preterm Birth from Infancy to Adulthood. *Lancet Lond. Engl.* **371**, 261–269 (2008).

100. Glass, H. C. *et al.* Outcomes for Extremely Premature Infants. *Anesth. Analg.* 120, 1337–1351 (2015).

101. Tyson, J. E. *et al.* Intensive Care for Extreme Prematurity - Moving Beyond Gestational Age. *N. Engl. J. Med.* **358**, 1672–1681 (2008).

102. Vincer, M. J. *et al.* Increasing Prevalence of Cerebral Palsy Among Very Preterm Infants: A Population-based Study. *Pediatrics* **118**, e1621–e1626 (2006).

103. Anderson, P., Doyle, L. W. and the Victorian Infant Collaborative Study Group. Neurobehavioral Outcomes of School-age Children Born Extremely Low Birth Weight or Very Preterm in the 1990s. *JAMA* **289**, 3264–3272 (2003).

104. Sykes, D. H. *et al.* Behavioural Adjustment in School of Very Low Birthweight Children. *J. Child Psychol. Psychiatry* **38**, 315–325 (1997).

105. Woodward, L. J., Anderson, P. J., Austin, N. C., Howard, K. & Inder, T. E. Neonatal MRI to Predict Neurodevelopmental Outcomes in Preterm Infants. *N. Engl. J. Med.* **355**, 685–694 (2006).

106. Chiswick, M. Infants of Borderline Viability: Ethical and Clinical Considerations. *Semin. Fetal. Neonatal Med.* **13**, 8–15 (2008).

107. Ancel, P.-Y. *et al.* Survival and Morbidity of Preterm Children Born at 22 Through 34 Weeks' Gestation in France in 2011: Results of the EPIPAGE-2 Cohort Study. *JAMA Pediatr.* **169**, 230–238 (2015).

108. Cheong, J. L. *et al.* Association Between Moderate and Late Preterm Birth and Neurodevelopment and Social-Emotional Development at Age 2 Years. *JAMA Pediatr.* **171**, e164805–e164805 (2017).

109. Srinivas Jois, R. Neurodevelopmental Outcome of Late-preterm infants: A Pragmatic Review. *Aust. J. Gen. Pract.* **47**, 776–781 (2018).

110. Shah, P., Kaciroti, N., Richards, B., Oh, W. & Lumeng, J. C. Developmental Outcomes of Late Preterm Infants From Infancy to Kindergarten. *Pediatrics* **138** (2016).

111. McGowan, J. E., Alderdice, F. A., Holmes, V. A. & Johnston, L. Early Childhood Development of Late-preterm Infants: A Systematic Review. *Pediatrics* 127, 1111–1124 (2011).

112. Agrawal, S., Rao, S. C., Bulsara, M. K. & Patole, S. K. Prevalence of Autism Spectrum Disorder in Preterm Infants: A Meta-analysis. *Pediatrics* 142, (2018).

113. Ben Itzchak, E., Lahat, E. & Zachor, D. A. Advanced Parental Ages and Low Birth Weight in Autism Spectrum Disorders – Rates and Effect on Functioning. *Res. Dev. Disabil.* 32, 1776–1781 (2011).

114. Maramara, L. A., He, W. & Ming, X. Pre- and Perinatal Risk Factors for Autism Spectrum Disorder in a New Jersey Cohort. *J. Child Neurol.* 29, 1645–1651 (2014).

115. Lampi, K. M. *et al.* Risk of Autism Spectrum Disorders in Low Birth Weight and Small for Gestational Age Infants. *J. Pediatr.* 161, 830–836 (2012).

116. Mann, J. R., McDermott, S., Bao, H., Hardin, J. & Gregg, A. Pre-eclampsia, Birth Weight, and Autism Spectrum Disorders. *J. Autism Dev. Disord.* 40, 548–554 (2010).

117. Russell, G., Rodgers, L. R., Ukoumunne, O. C. & Ford, T. Prevalence of Parent-Reported ASD and ADHD in the UK: Findings from the Millennium Cohort Study. *J. Autism Dev. Disord.* 1–10 (2013). doi:10.1007/s10803-013-1849-0

118. Salmaso, N., Jablonska, B., Scafidi, J., Vaccarino, F. M. & Gallo, V. Neurobiology of Premature Brain Injury. *Nat. Neurosci.* 17, 341–346 (2014).

119. de Haan, M. *et al.* Brain and Cognitive-behavioural Development After Asphyxia at Term Birth. *Dev. Sci.* 9, 350–358 (2006).

120. Verhaeghe, L. *et al.* Extremely Preterm Born Children at Very High Risk for Developing Autism Spectrum Disorder. *Child Psychiatry Hum. Dev.* 47, 729–739 (2016). doi:10.1007/s10578-015-0606-3.

121. Lampi, K. M. *et al.* Risk of Autism Spectrum Disorders in Low Birth Weight and Small for Gestational Age Infants. *J. Pediatr.* 161, 830–836 (2012).

122. Guy, A. *et al.* Infants Born Late/Moderately Preterm Are at Increased Risk for a Positive Autism Screen at 2 Years of Age. *J. Pediatr.* 166, 269–275.e3 (2015).

123. Keyes, K. M. *et al.* Cohort Effects Explain the Increase in Autism Diagnosis Among Children Born from 1992 to 2003 in California. *Int. J. Epidemiol.* 41, 495–503 (2012).

124. Kukla, R. Pregnant Bodies as Public Spaces. In *Motherhood and Space: Configurations of the Maternal Through Politics, Home, and the Body* (eds. Hardy, S. & Wiedmer, C.) 283–305 (Palgrave Macmillan US, 2005). doi:10.1007/978-1-137-12103-5_16.

125. Modabbernia, A., Velthorst, E. & Reichenberg, A. Environmental Risk Factors for Autism: An Evidence-based Review of Systematic Reviews and Meta-analyses. *Mol. Autism* 8(13) (2017) eCollection 2017.

126. Zhang, B. *et al.* Inflammatory Bowel Disease is Associated with Higher Dementia Risk: A Nationwide Longitudinal Study. *Gut* (2020) doi:10.1136/gutjnl-2020-320789.

127. Newschaffer, C. J. *et al.* The Epidemiology of Autism Spectrum Disorders. *Annu. Rev. Public Health* 28, 235–258 (2007).

128. Newschaffer, C. J., Fallin, D. & Lee, N. L. Heritable and Nonheritable Risk Factors for Autism Spectrum Disorders. *Epidemiol. Rev.* 24, 137–153 (2002).

129. Jiang, H.-Y. *et al.* Maternal Infection During Pregnancy and Risk of Autism Spectrum Disorders: A Systematic Review and Meta-analysis. *Brain. Behav. Immun.* 58, 165–172 (2016).

130. Wolke, D. *et al.* Selective Drop-out in Longitudinal Studies and Non-biased Prediction of Behaviour Disorders. *Br. J. Psychiatry* **195**, 249–256 (2009).
131. Yang, S. *et al.* Trends on $PM_{2.5}$ Research, 1997–2016: A Bibliometric Study. *Environ. Sci. Pollut. Res.* **25**, 12284–12298 (2018).
132. Singh, J., Illes, J., Lazzeroni, L. & Hallmayer, J. Trends in US Autism Research Funding. *J. Autism Dev. Disord.* **39**, 788–795 (2009).
133. Hacking, I. Inaugural Lecture: Chair of Philosophy and History of Scientific Concepts at the Collège de France, 16 January 2001. *Econ. Soc.* **31**, 1–14 (2002).

9 Factors during infancy, childhood and adulthood

Exacerbation

This chapter contemplates the psycho-social and environmental factors that exacerbate or provoke the 'symptoms' of autism (in other words, the behaviours that qualify as autistic). Although these are not plausible as reasons to explain the rise in autism diagnosis, the outcome (more autistic behaviours) is the same. I tentatively suggest that these factors are best described as exacerbations rather than risks, because their effects are more transient. They are also more accurately described as exacerbators or as provoking autistic behaviour, while autism is understood as originating in neurological difference, which is fixed at birth. Within the constraints of this framework of understanding autism, environmental exposures after infancy can only intensify pre-existing autism, rather than instigate it. However, this distinction takes work to police, as studies of psycho-social deprivation have shown.

Psycho-social deprivation

An estimated 100,000 Romanian children were living in orphanages at the end of 1989, after the fall of the Ceauşescu regime. Many of the children were not orphans but their parents could not afford large families, and abortions and contraception were banned. Conditions in orphanages were dreadful; the electricity supply and heating were intermittent and food was in short supply.[1] The worst circumstances were found in children's psychiatric hospitals, which lacked washing facilities, and where the bodily and sexual abuse of children was reportedly commonplace.[2] Children were often restrained, tied to their beds by their own clothes. Sometimes children were left lying in their own urine. Many had delayed cognitive development and did not know how to feed themselves.[2]

Infants continued to enter the orphanages after the fall of Ceauşescu.[2] Throughout the 1990s, thousands of infants in Romanian care settings had almost no physical contact with caregivers. Psycho-social deprivation – basically little or no stimulation and negligible human contact – was rife. The babies had cots, were fed and had their soiled nappies changed. But in many cases, there was almost no relationship forming and nurturing. Improving the orphanages was a condition of Romania's entry to the European Union in 2007 but the BBC journalist, Chris Rogers, reported in 2009 that conditions in some institutions were still very poor.

Michael Rutter and colleagues spent several decades studying the 'English Romanian adoptees', a group of 165 Romanian children who were institutionalised as infants but adopted by families in the UK. Rutter wanted to determine the effects of early psycho-social deprivation on the Romanian infants, using measures such as social difficulties and repetitive behaviours.[3] Compared to a control group of adopted children born in the UK, his team found a very high incidence of these autistic behaviours in the cohort of institutionalised Romanian children when they were four to six years old, even after their adoption by families in the UK.[4]

Another study, again led by Rutter, followed the same children into adolescence but only sampled among those with an intelligence quotient (IQ) of at least 50. This study again found a high level of autistic-type behaviours in the Romanian-born children (just under 10% of the Romanian adoptees), as opposed to none in the UK-born adoptees.[3] An additional 6% of the Romanian adoptees had milder autistic-like 'features'. By the age of 11, the severity of the autistic-type behaviours had diminished but not completely disappeared; a quarter of the Romanian children adopted into the UK no longer had autistic behaviour. However, for the rest, many autistic-type behaviours persisted into adolescence.[5]

This study also compared the Romanian adoptees who had spent less than six months in an institution with those who spent more than six months there.[5] The differences between the Romanian group that had been institutionalised for less than six months and the UK-born adoptees were negligible on a range of neurodevelopmental and cognitive measures. By contrast, the group with longer exposure to the institutional setting displayed higher rates of autism-type behaviours, including disinhibition, poor social skills, inattention and hyperactivity, even as young adults.[5] This group also had higher rates of cognitive impairment, low educational achievement, unemployment and higher use of mental health services in adulthood.[5] This finding suggests that children's autistic-type and attention deficit hyperactivity disorder (ADHD)-type outcomes might be determined by the length and timing of their exposure to severe neglect in infancy.

The Bucharest Early Intervention Project followed a second cohort of Romanian institutionally raised children, who were randomly allocated either to good-quality family foster care or to continue in institutional care.[6] Again, high levels of autistic behaviours were observed. Roughly 60% of the children demonstrated repetitive movements or sounds at around two years old (although such behaviours are common in all infants). These behaviours were eased but not erased as they matured; more so for those placed with foster families.[7] The lucky group placed with family foster carers also had better social communication skills, compared to the comparison group who remained in institutions. About 5% of the children continued to meet the criteria for autism irrespective of whether they moved to foster care.[8] Adoptees often continued to exhibit social disinhibition (such as hugging strangers), regardless of which group they were placed in.[8]

Autism-type behaviours, the authors of both sets of studies surmised, were most probably rooted in the children's early lack of social experience. They argued there is a critical window for development in infancy – a time when nurture is crucial for normal neurodevelopment.[5] During the first two years, babies' basic nurturing and contact needs must be met if behaviours reminiscent of autism and ADHD are not to be aggravated. But note the language: 'reminiscent of'.

Quasi-autism

Rutter and his group argued that the Romanian orphans who were diagnosed with autism probably do not have the same condition as others with autism. They called it 'quasi-autism'.[3] The 'quasi' distinction hung on the account of the adoptees having slightly different features from true autism: disinhibited attachment, more flexible (albeit unusual) communication styles and improvements in some as they matured. A disproportionate number of adoptees 'lost' the diagnosis as they got older.

The 'quasi-' designation was given despite the adoptees meeting existing autism diagnostic criteria and the enormous heterogeneity of current understandings of autism, the diagnosis of which can encompass the disinhibited social behaviour and abnormal but flexible communication described as distinctive in the quasi-autism group. Moreover, all children with autistic traits have different trajectories and some, but not others, mature to sub-clinical levels.[9–12] For all these reasons, it takes work to distinguish the quasi- from the true.

The distinction was needed to maintain (and enhance) the integrity of 'true' autism as it was – and is – understood: a lifelong condition that is normally present from birth. The authors made the argument that what they witnessed was not actually autism, meaning that deprivation can't possibly trigger 'true' autism. The adoptees' autistic-like traits were expressed due to neglect, not because of inborn neurodevelopmental difference. 'Quasi-autism' is prominent in this seminal article's title.[3] Rutter and his colleagues emphasised that the adoptees' symptoms, especially the 11-year-old children's difficulties in picking up social cues, only resembled autism-as-we-know-it. Moreover, the article's first line, 'despite the evidence that autism constitutes a disorder that is strongly influenced by genetic factors', emphasises the biological aetiology of true autism.[3]

However, most of the Romanian adoptees *did not* have autism-type behaviours. This suggests that the sub-section of adoptees who developed autistic behaviours had a genetic predisposition to do so; that their autistic-type behaviours stemmed from a combination of genetics and early institutional deprivation. To distinguish the quasi- from the true on the basis of aetiology seems harder work when both have a biological basis.

Work on children's general neurological development has shown that maltreatment alters the trajectories of brain development. Early deprivation and later abuse may have effects on amygdala volume.[13] Structural and functional neurological abnormalities initially attributed to innate conditions may be a more direct consequence of neglect and abuse. These brain changes may be thought to be best understood as adaptive responses to enable endurance in the face of adversity.[13] Childhood maltreatment is the most important preventable cause of psychopathology, accounting for about 45% of the attributable risk for childhood-onset psychiatric disorders such as depression, anxiety, substance abuse, eating disorders, suicidal symptomatology, psychosis and personality disorder. But this list omits autism.[13]

The idea that autism always occurs from birth (except in rare cases of regressive autism) is extremely useful and does great work for the various tribes, thus ensuring it is worth policing. 'Born this way' has been proclaimed by autistic awareness activists,[14] who have compellingly argued that autism is, was and ever will be an unchangeable part of themselves.[15] Autism is a fundamental difference in 'wiring' that can't be reversed, therefore society needs to shift and accommodate. This strong and persuasive argument for disability rights renders unpalatable the idea that autism might only become apparent due to an infant or child's environment.[16]

A second form of reason for invoking the 'quasi-' qualifier is the fear of a return to the abysmal refrigerator mother theory described by Bruno Bettelheim in his book *The Empty Fortress*, published in the 1960s.[17] The history and emergence of this theory, loosely aligned with John Bowlby's attachment theory, are described in great depth in various texts.[18–20] Briefly, mothers were blamed for their children's autism, which was thought to be a consequence of cold and inadequate parenting. The idea did untold damage, resulting in blaming, stigmatising and attribution of guilt to mothers (a tradition which continues in parenting). To heal the effects of this alleged psycho-social derivation, holding therapy involved the carer forcefully holding the child until the child 'surrendered' and looked into the carer's eyes, even against their will.[21] The suggestion of reviving the 'refrigerator' is chilling. Rutter himself was instrumental in demonstrating the high heritability of autistic traits, estimating that heritability was as high as 90%, with little contribution from the environment.[22, 23] In the 1990s, this led to autism's healthy re-construction as one of the most heritable of all psychiatric conditions, as opposed to primarily being a disorder of attachment, whereas the Romanian orphans clearly suffered from lack of attachment to nurturing parents.[24]

Autism-as-innate is a far kinder understanding of autism and one less stigmatising of parents. The rise of biological psychiatry and cognitive psychology, which became dominant over psychoanalytic models in the 1990s, saw a welcome shift in conceptualisation to a difference in cognitive processing, located in neural mechanisms, underpinned by a strong genetic component.[25] This neurological, geneticised framework has become somewhat reified, in part because of the work it does in protecting parents who refuse to be blamed, biologically minded scientists who seek a pharmacological treatment and self-advocates who argue for rights and accommodations.[26] Writing about medically unexplained symptoms, Monica Greco argues it suits all parties to minimise any possibility of a psychological aetiology.[27]

A similar device to 'quasi-' has been used to position adult-onset ADHD, a phenomenon only recently discovered. Researchers have argued that, although adults with adult-onset ADHD show behaviours (symptoms) indistinguishable from true ADHD, it is in fact a different condition.[28] Adult-onset ADHD 'is a *bona fide* disorder that has unfortunately been mistaken for the neurodevelopmental disorder of ADHD because of surface similarities and given the wrong name'.[29] Like autism, ADHD is thought of as neurodevelopmental, with a strong genetic component and onset in childhood. To defend the existing model of ADHD, the adult-onset version cannot be 'true'. Recall, however, Rutter's words of wisdom: our definitions of disorder are ever-changing, pragmatic attempts to group behavioural traits that cause distress. In his eyes, there is no 'true' autism or ADHD, only useful models worth defending.

The Romanian cohort studies also raise the question of whether only very severe neglect in infancy gives rise to the kind of autistic and ADHD traits seen in the Romanian adoptees, or whether milder cases of neglect also prompt perhaps less-pronounced differences in neurodevelopment. In other words, is it risk accumulation (such as neglect suffered in childhood in combination with environmental and genetic risk factors) or only very specific risk exposure (such as very severe neglect lasting more than six months) that shapes neurodevelopmental and cognitive outcomes?

In the USA, in common with other high-income countries, maltreatment is highest in children aged between new-born and three years old but rates of child maltreatment have dropped.[30] In the UK, data suggest cases of infant neglect and entry into care have increased since 1990.[31] Thankfully, however, the mass and very severe institutional deprivation witnessed in Romania has not been replicated elsewhere, making infant neglect implausible as any kind of trigger for the observed rise in autism diagnoses.

A study of stimming

During childhood, environmental and social stimuli can further exacerbate behaviours charcteristic of autism. Autism affects how children interact and communicate in the social realm. But autism can also affect a child's relationship with their environment and this can result in modified behaviour, such as repetitive movements or an intense desire for sameness. These latter features form part of the so-called 'non-social features' of the fifth edition of the *Diagnostic and Statistical Manual of Mental Disorders* (DSM-5) diagnostic criteria for autism. Repetitive movements such as hand flapping are known among autistics as 'stimming' (a contraction of self-stimulating).

There is an important distinction in developmental psychology between traits and states. A trait is a more enduring characteristic than a state. A state is transient, often triggering the onset of specific behaviour. The psychologist Richard Bentall points out that psychological characteristics vary from being trait-like and immutable to being state-like and changeable.[32] He further describes the concept of a spectrum that extends into the normal and sub-clinical range as the 'principle of continuity', asserting that:

> *Abnormal behaviours and experiences are related to normal behaviours by continua of frequency (the same behaviours and experiences occur less frequently*

in non-psychiatric populations), severity (less severe forms of behaviour and experiences can be identified in non-psychiatric populations) and phenomenology (non-clinical analogues of behaviour can be identified as part of normal life).[32]

As discussed, the imposition of a cut-off between abnormality and normality, diagnosis or no diagnosis, is therefore an arbitrary but convenient way of converting a dimension into a category, as Robert Goodman and Stephen Scott point out in their textbook of child psychiatry.[33] Charles Nelson, the co-lead of the Bucharest adoptees' study, noted that the Romanian infants, who lacked external stimulation, often resorted to self-stimulation. Instances of self-stimulation induced by the severely neglectful circumstances of the infants held 'captive' in the orphanages included hand flapping or rocking. Stimming, or in psycho-parlance 'stereotypic behaviour', is defined as being repetitive, unvarying and with no apparent goal or function, and is seen in laboratory, farm and zoo mammals.[34] Behaviours observed in laboratory monkeys and primates that have been separated from their mothers at birth or in the first year of life and brought up in partial or total social isolation include rocking, huddling, self-abuse and sucking.[35] Animal studies show confinement in infancy may have a permanent effect on the infant animal's ability to interact in a flexible and creative way with its environment, analogous with the quasi-autistic behaviour observed in the Romanian children. The emphasis in animal studies is on the permanence of these behaviours, suggesting that the environment of infancy can enduringly affect the way in which the nervous system develops.[36] In adoptee studies, although some autistic behaviour endured, the emphasis was generally put on improvements in foster care.

In psychology, behaviour that represents a restriction of behavioural possibilities is described as 'perseverative'.[36] Perseverative behaviour includes restricted interests or insistence on sameness but can also include repeated behaviours, such as taking the same route each day or always organising food on a plate in the same manner. Both are seen in the non-psychiatric populations that Bentall's principle describes, albeit at lower frequencies and severity it is good to recall, too, that the boundaries of what is considered psychiatric and what is non psychiatric changes with time and circumstances, and is subject to lobbying.

There is a disparity between how the scientific and broader autism communities view and describe the so-called stereotypic, repetitive behaviours. Rocking, hand flapping and finger flicking are all forms of stimming that appear in the diagnostic criteria for autism. Having conducted several interviews in which autistic adults spoke about stimming, I was aghast at how stimming seemed to be viewed so differently in scientific circles than by those who actually do it. The autistic community has reclaimed and actively supports 'stimming', originally a derogatory word.[37] To help adjust the balance, we conducted a study to examine autistic adults' accounts of how and why they stim and what stimming means to them.[38]

The autistic experience is so varied that we did not attempt to try and capture everything; that would be impossible. But one of the aims of our study was to change the conversation from looking at stimming, repetitive and restricted behaviours as a 'behavioural symptom' to consideration of the diverse experience of the stimmers and their reasons for stimming. I approached Liz Pellicano, who introduced me to Robyn Steward, an autistic advocate, educator, researcher and musician, who had already conducted a survey on the topic of stimming among the autism community.[39] Steward's online survey reported that 50% of autistic people said they enjoyed stimming, yet 72% had been told not to do it. Many (58%) stimmed when *over*stimulated; the most commonly cited reasons for stimming were to reduce anxiety (72%) or to calm down (69%).

We decided to run a series of workshops to ask adults about their experiences. There was a good deal of additional interview data with autistic adults, and further interview snippets are quoted here. To include autistic adults with a diverse range of needs, we recruited adults with high support needs living in two residential homes as well as people living in other settings.

Overstimulating environments

Our participants told us that environmental triggers such as artificial lighting, crowded and confusing social environments full of activity, exposure to loud or unpleasant sounds, strong odours and uncomfortable temperatures or substrates made autistic people uncomfortable and anxious and provoked bouts of stimming. Distressing social environments included confinement-specific stressors such as restricted movement, reduced retreat space, forced proximity to others and unfamiliar social groups. For example, one participant described a stim-provoking visit to a 'restaurant [with], lot of sensory information going on'. My previous job, pre PhD, having been as a television producer, this description reminded me of a film set, with much activity and many lights, cameras and new people to negotiate, all in an inescapable work environment.

Stimming could engender a sense of control and restore balance. According to one participant stimming was 'performing an action or vocalisation, often rhythmic in some way, to help oneself cope with a stressful situation. So rocking, humming, flapping hands kind of thing'. Equally, stimming was used to express intense joy and respond to a heightened positive emotional state. Another participant stated that 'stimming to me is a natural expression of joy, excitement, anxiety and worries but also a strategy that helps my body process my thoughts, feelings and energies'. Stimming seems to be a way for people to regulate over-powering emotions, be they negative or positive.

The types of exposures reported to trigger stereotypies in animal studies include environmental sources of stress such as artificial lighting and exposure to brash or aversive noises, extreme temperatures or sensory stimuli or an unvarying environment.[40] We cannot equate autistic adults with captive animals but the animal studies underline the point that proximal environmental triggers can and do precipitate stereotypies or stims. 'All people and some mammals stim. Autistic people do it more because we exist in a world where there's a poor person–environment fit. Society is designed for neurotypical people', as one participant put it.

Stims can be what diagnostic criteria describe as 'symptoms' but they seem to have a useful calming function according to the testimony we heard: 'has the calming effect', 'to help oneself cope with a stressful situation', 'stimming can prevent you getting into an anxious state'. But, just as importantly, stimming was also likely to be provoked by extreme joy and overwhelming happiness: 'thinking about exciting racing … I was making like funny like movements'. Anyone who has seen a toddler waving their hands in glee and excitement can appreciate that stims can be expressive of either anxiety or joy. Our study built on Steward's work, and participants' testimony backed up the idea that stims can be a useful way to regulate emotion, an idea that has been put forward before, although approached in a new way.[41] I devised an initial simple model (Figure 9.1) which Steven Kapp developed into a more comprehensive picture for publication.

A second finding, not yet published, was that allistic people also frequently found themselves 'stimming': tapping a foot, pulling hair, joggling legs, drumming fingers. Although the difference was unclear, they often did not call it 'stimming' but rather 'fidgeting'. Stimming seems to be a pursuit that all people take part in, to a greater or lesser extent, but perhaps name differently because of the severity and frequency, and perhaps phenomenology, as in Bentall's descriptions of clinical versus non-clinical behaviour. This is a line of enquiry Kapp hopes to follow in future analysis of the dataset.

Participants described how their stimming was deemed unacceptable in public, and some private, spaces. Some autism interventions have aimed to minimise stimming; recent articles have summarised interventions aimed at minimising restricted and repetitive behaviours.[42] If stimming plays a useful function, and is harmless, this seems a ludicrous ambition. 'How would I calm down [if stimming were suppressed]?' asked one participant. 'If you're taking away someone's ability

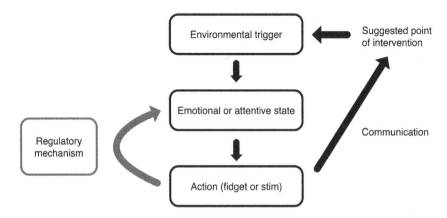

Figure 9.1 An initial model of stimming as regulatory mechanism.

to cope in a situation, when they're in that situation I worry they are going to have a breakdown'. Another described how for her, stimming had become a way to self-regulate her emotions: 'I never used to wave my hands that much but I've started doing it more, it actually helps ... which is quite incredible'. Some scholars argue that Applied Behaviour Analysis (ABA), a well-used behavioural intervention, has sometimes been used to force autistics to comply in ways that are actively damaging and do little to bring about acceptance. Indeed, they argue, this makes society worse, by reinforcing the stigmatisation of autistic behaviours. In response to the suggestion that a reduction in stimming may reduce the bullying of the stimmer, it is noted that bullying is aberrant behaviour and that the person in need of a behavioural intervention is the bully. It is paradoxical that our societal norms and interventions stigmatise by rewarding suppression of autistic stims. We argued the site of intervention, if any is required, should be the environment, not the individual child (Figure 9.1).

The broadening of the spectrum to include cognitively able children means many more children with diagnosed autism are now in mainstream schools. I wonder if behaviours teachers called 'fidgeting' in former times are now classed as autistic 'symptoms' of diagnosed pupils. In an earlier study, I listened to parents talk of children's meltdowns and bouts of stimming on arriving home, prompted by holding it together at secondary schools in which 'autistic' behaviours were stigmatising. One participant noted that, although stimming was tolerated in younger children, such tolerance decreased with age. Perhaps acceptance and understanding of the ameliorating function of stimming is one key to neurodiversity awareness in schools.[41]

To summarise, while behavioural science describes stereotypies in humans (and other mammals), autistic people describe stims. While some behavioural interventions try to dampen stereotypies, autistic people regard stims as helpful and encourage them. The autistic anthology *Loud Hands* is a response to the command, 'quiet hands'. Keep still, don't stim.[43] If the built and captive environments trigger anxiety and distress in animals and humans we should work to change the environments, not the living creatures.

To return to the main question, could changes to the built and social environment have elicited more stimming and other autistic behaviours since 1990, leading to more identification of autism? Are schools, for example, more crowded and difficult to navigate? This seems highly debatable, as autistic behaviours must be pervasive across multiple settings, for example both at home and school, to qualify for diagnosis.

Traits versus states

My far-from-comprehensive review of risks and exacerbating factors in Part II was organised by life stages. One tentative conclusion is that the earlier in the life course a risk is encountered, the more trait-like and less state-like the resulting autistic behaviours appear to be. Environmental or social risks at very early stages

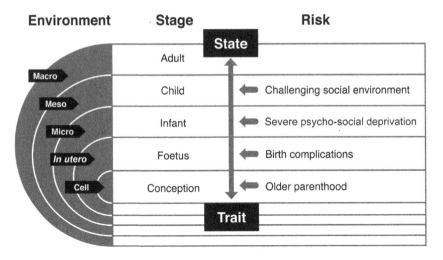

Figure 9.2 Antecedents of autistic behavioural states versus autistic traits.

of development seem to produce more trait-like results, whereas later influences exacerbate or provoke more transient behavioural states (Figure 9.2).

In reality, the frequency, severity and pervasiveness of particular behaviours are considered when diagnosing autism, as well as their persistence. But the state/trait divide may be a useful way to conceptualise risk across the life course. On the one hand, older parenthood, which can disturb the quality of the gametes and the meiotic replication of DNA at conception, seems to be associated with more permanent and core autistic traits. Hypoxia at birth can give rise to severe and permanent brain damage. On the other hand, the early severe psycho-social deprivation experienced by Romanian infants resulted in autistic-type behaviours that were often (but not always) ameliorated when they were placed with foster families, and encountering unwelcome social environments in adulthood triggered transient bouts of stimming states.

Figure 9.2 draws on Urie Bronfenbrenner's ecological systems theory of child development, which centres a child among layers of influence that shape the child's adaptation to their environment.[44] In Bronfenbrenner's model, the macro-level environment is the surrounding socio-cultural environment; the meso-level the culture of the child's neighbourhood and community; and the micro-level the child's family and direct caregivers, such as teachers and babysitters. As children grow and develop, they reach out from their existing level of understanding and experience to increasingly wider spheres. Smaller layers can be added, in ever-decreasing circles, through foetal development (the *in utero* environment) to conception (the development of the genome in the cellular environment).

In later work, Bronfenbrenner emphasised bi-directional effects; the individual person is both shaped by and shapes their environment.[45] Bi-directional effects seem more and more pertinent as life progresses and the child grows more independent from the parent. A blastocyst has no conscious control over its uterine environment, a child a little control over its, an adult most control of all. Maturing means following a path to independence, autonomy and the resilience to bring up one's own offspring. The earlier in the lifespan a threat occurs, the more vulnerable the person is to those threats.

Threats, considered as risk factors associated with neurodevelopment or neural processes, can also operate at each stage; human neural development adapts and responds to the environment at every stage of the lifespan. The effects of environmental risks on neurodevelopment seem to have more impact and last longer if they occur in the fragile early stages (moderated by the severity of the risk). This temporality of response to environmental risk factors, more trait-like for early risks and more state-like for later meso- and macro-level risks, seems to be aligned to the age at which the factor is experienced and level of biology in operation (Figure 9.2). The environments of earlier stages seem more influential than later stages in determining the permanence of autistic traits. Later environments, such as school, that are more associated with behavioural states, are better considered as exacerbating factors rather than risks.

State/trait theory fits with the idea of the critical developmental window, the closure of which means the opportunity to ameliorate the difficulties of the child will be lost. Window thinking can be used as a prompt for early detection, diagnosis and intervention, which fits with conventional wisdom on early intervention. But science, as discussed earlier, can be good at telling the stories the discipline wants to hear. My states/traits diagram is best thought of as tentative and a potential area for further research, rather than a claim of knowledge.

References

1. Steavenson, W. Ceausescu's Children. *The Guardian* (2014).
2. BBC News Channel. Our World, Ceausescu's Children. www.bbc.co.uk/programmes/b00qby76. (2010).
3. Rutter, M. *et al.* Early Adolescent Outcomes of Institutionally Deprived and Non-deprived Adoptees. III. Quasi-autism. *J. Child Psychol. Psychiatry* **48**, 1200–1207 (2007).
4. Rutter, M. *et al.* Quasi-autistic Patterns Following Severe Early Global Privation. English and Romanian Adoptees (ERA) Study Team. *J. Child Psychol. Psychiatry* **40**, 537–549 (1999).
5. Sonuga-Barke, E. J. S. *et al.* Child-to-adult Neurodevelopmental and Mental Health Trajectories After Early Life Deprivation: The Young Adult Follow-up of the Longitudinal English and Romanian Adoptees Study. *Lancet Lond. Engl.* **389**, 1539–1548 (2017).
6. Levin, A. R., Fox, N. A., Zeanah, C. H. & Nelson, C. A. Social Communication Difficulties and Autism in Previously Institutionalized Children. *J. Am. Acad. Child Adolesc. Psychiatry* **54**, 108–115.e1 (2015).
7. Bos, K. J., Zeanah, C. H., Smyke, A. T., Fox, N. A. & Nelson, C. A. Stereotypies in Children with a History of Early Institutional Care. *Arch. Pediatr. Adolesc. Med.* **164**, 406–411 (2010).

8. Romanian Orphans Reveal Clues to Origins of Autism. *Spectrum | Autism Research News* www.spectrumnews.org/opinion/viewpoint/romanian-orphans-reveal-clues-origins-autism/ (2017).

9. Russell, G. *et al.* Social and Behavioural Outcomes in Children Diagnosed with Autism Spectrum Disorders: A Longitudinal Cohort Study. *J. Child Psychol. Psychiatry* **53**, 735–744 (2012).

10. Baghdadli, A. *et al.* Developmental Trajectories of Adaptive Behaviors from Early Childhood to Adolescence in a Cohort of 152 Children with Autism Spectrum Disorders. *J. Autism Dev. Disord.* **42**, 1314–1325 (2012).

11. Szatmari, P. *et al.* Similar Developmental Trajectories in Autism and Asperger Syndrome: From Early Childhood to Adolescence. *J. Child Psychol. Psychiatry* **50**, 1459–1467 (2009).

12. Turner, L. M. & Stone, W. L. Variability in Outcome for Children with an ASD Diagnosis at Age 2. *J. Child Psychol. Psychiatry* **48**, 793–802 (2007).

13. Teicher, M. H. & Samson, J. A. Annual Research Review: Enduring Neurobiological Effects of Childhood Abuse and Neglect. *J. Child Psychol. Psychiatry* **57**, 241–266 (2016).

14. *Autism- Born This Way.* www.youtube.com/watch?v=YC_MY9vMV0U (2020).

15. Sinclair, J. Why I Dislike 'Person First' Language. *Auton. Crit. J. Interdiscip. Autism Stud.* **1**, (2013).

16. Russell, G. Critiques of the Neurodiversity Movement. In *Autistic Community and the Neurodiversity Movement: Stories from the Frontline* (ed. Kapp, S. K.) 287–303 (Springer, 2020). doi:10.1007/978-981-13-8437-0_21

17. Bettelheim, B. *The Empty Fortress.* (Free Press, 1972).

18. Nadesan, M. *Constructing Autism: Unravelling the 'Truth' and Understanding the Social* (Routledge, 2005).

19. Waltz, M. *Autism: A Social and Medical History* (Palgrave Macmillan, 2013).

20. Silberman, S. *Neurotribes: The Legacy of Autism and How to Think Smarter About People Who Think Differently* (Allen & Unwin, 2015).

21. *Enhancing Early Attachments: Theory, Research, Intervention, and Policy.* xxiv, 357 (Guilford Press, 2005).

22. Folstein, S. & Rutter, M. Infantile Autism: A Genetic Study of 21 Twin Pairs. *J. Child Psychol. Psychiatry* **18**, 297–321 (1977).

23. Bailey, A. *et al.* Autism as a Strongly Genetic Disorder: Evidence from a British Twin Study. *Psychol. Med.* **25**, 63–77 (1995).

24. Yuen, R.K.C. Szatmari, P. & Vorstman, J. A. S., M. B. The Genetics of Autism Spectrum Disorders. In *Autism and Pervasive Developmental Disorders* (Cambridge University Press, 2019) p 112–129.

25. Smith, M. *Hyperactive: A History of ADHD* (Reaktion Books, 2012).

26. Silverman, C. & Brosco, J. P. Understanding Autism: Parents and Pediatricians in Historical Perspective. *Arch. Pediatr. Adolesc. Med.* **161**, 392–398 (2007).

27. Greco, M. The Classification and Nomenclature of 'Medically Unexplained Symptoms': Conflict, Performativity and Critique. *Soc. Sci. Med.* **75**, 2362–2369 (2012).

28. Castellanos, F. X. Is Adult-onset ADHD a Distinct Entity? *Am. J. Psychiatry* **172**, 929–931 (2015).

29. Moffitt, T. E. *et al.* Is Adult ADHD a Childhood-onset Neurodevelopmental Disorder? Evidence From a Four-decade Longitudinal Cohort Study. *Am. J. Psychiatry* **172**, 967–977 (2015).

30. Child Maltreatment. *Child Trends* www.childtrends.org/indicators/child-maltreatment.

31. Esposti, M. D. *et al.* Long-term Trends in Child Maltreatment in England and Wales, 1858–2016: An Observational, Time-series Analysis. *Lancet Public Health* 4, e148–e158 (2019).

32. Bentall, R. P. *Madness Explained: Psychosis and Human Nature* (Penguin Books Ltd, 2004).

33. Goodman, R. & Scott, S. *Child Psychiatry* (Blackwell Publishing, 1997).

34. Latham, N. R. & Mason, G. J. Maternal Deprivation and the Development of Stereotypic Behaviour. *Appl. Anim. Behav. Sci.* 110, 84–108 (2008).

35. Animal Welfare Institute. *Towards an Understanding of Stereotypic Behaviour in Laboratory Macaques.* www.awionline.org/content/towards-understanding-stereotypic-behaviour-laboratory-macaques (2020).

36. Ridley, R. M. The Psychology of Perseverative and Stereotyped Behaviour. *Prog. Neurobiol.* 44, 221–231 (1994).

37. Nolan, J. & McBride, M. Embodied Semiosis: Autistic 'Stimming' as Sensory Praxis. In *International Handbook of Semiotics* (ed. Trifonas, P. P.) 1069–1078 (Springer, Dordrecht, 2015). doi:10.1007/978-94-017-9404-6_48.

38. Kapp, S. K., Steward, R., Crane, L., Elliott, D., Elphick, C., Pellicano, L. & Russell, G. People Should be Allowed to do what they Like: Autistic Adults' Views and Experiences of Stimming. *Autism* 1362361319829628 (2019). https://doi.org/10.1177/1362361319829628

39. Steward, R. L. Repetitive Stereotyped Behaviour or 'Stimming': An Online Survey of 100 People on the Autism Spectrum. https://insar.confex.com/insar/2015/webprogram/Paper20115.html (2015).

40. Mason, G. Stereotypic Behaviour in Captive Animals: Fundamentals and Implications for Welfare and Beyond. In *Stereotypic Animal Behaviour: Fundamentals and Applications to Welfare* (eds. Mason, G. & Rushen, J.) 325–356 (CABI, 2006). doi:10.1079/9780851990040.0325

41. Leekam, S. R., Prior, M. R. & Uljarevic, M. Restricted and Repetitive Behaviours in Autism Spectrum Disorders: A Review of Research in the Last Decade. *Psychol. Bull.* 137, 562–593 (2011).

42. Boyd, B. A., McDonough, S. G. & Bodfish, J. W. Evidence-based Behavioral Interventions for Repetitive Behaviors in Autism. *J. Autism Dev. Disord.* 42, 1236–1248 (2012).

43. Bascom, J. *Loud Hands: Autistic People, Speaking* (Autistic Press, 2012).

44. Bronfenbrenner, U. *The Ecology of Human Development: Experiments by Nature and Design* (Harvard University Press, 1979).

45. Bronfenbrenner, U. & Ceci, S. J. Nature–nurture Reconceptualized in Developmental Perspective: A Bioecological Model. *Psychol. Rev.* 101, 568–586 (1994).

10 Diagnosis

Assessing diagnosis

In medicine, the value of diagnoses are assessed in terms of their validity, clinical utility and reliability.[1] A diagnosis is said to be *valid* if it measures the construct it is supposed to and reflects reality; that is, it is a class that 'carves nature at the joints'. It is *reliable* if the same diagnosis is given repeatedly by different clinicians in different settings, a skill that can be trained.[2] And it is *clinically useful* if it predicts needs and prospects, is a useful communication tool and can be used to prescribe effective treatment in the clinic.

The validity of all diagnoses in the fifth edition of the *Diagnostic and Statistical Manual of Mental Disorders* (DSM-5) has been challenged in ways covered in this book, using autism as a case in point. First, the validity of autism has been questioned because autism never occurs in isolation but almost always with other neurodevelopmental issues. This has led researchers to call for a 'lumping' of the category into a larger overarching neurodevelopmental framework. Groups such as Chris Gillberg's argue that, to better reflect reality in clinical practice, the gamut of neurodevelopmental disorders that present with impairing behaviours in childhood, including attention deficit hyperactivity disorder (ADHD), autism spectrum disorder (ASD), developmental co-ordination disorder, intellectual disability, speech and language impairment, dyslexia, dyspraxia, Tourette syndrome, early-onset bipolar disorder, behaviour phenotype syndromes and neurological and seizure disorders, should be lumped together as ESSENCE (early symptomatic syndromes eliciting neurodevelopmental clinical examinations).[3] Gillberg's team points out that, for developmental disorders, co-morbidity is the rule, not the exception.[3]

Second, the validity of autism diagnosis is challenged because autism is not a characteristic of an individual person but may become problematic only in relation to the social context (Chapter 9), because diagnosis converts a continuum of traits in the population to a binary (Chapter 4) and because autism is now so heterogeneous that there are multiple aetiological pathways that do not hang together if nosology is based on underlying pathology (Chapter 3). Because of these concerns over validity,[4] people have suggested 'splitting' by sub-types. In the case of autism, there may be 'multiple autisms', perhaps by genetic profiles,

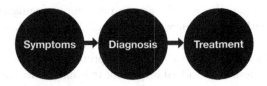

Figure 10.1 Simple medical model of clinical diagnosis.

cognitive profiles, neural differences, intellectual ability, gender or sensory processing differences. There are calls too to split autism research into studies of different types of traits.[5]

A traditional, medical, view of diagnosis is equivalent to a mechanic diagnosing why a car engine won't start. The symptom (the engine won't start) is due to a mechanical fault (the spark plugs are degraded). The mechanic identifies the fault (diagnosis) and implements a treatment (replacing the plugs) that solves the problem (Figure 10.1). The validity of the diagnostic category is further eroded by the presumed neutrality of diagnosis in this model (which nobody really subscribes to); a diagnosis is supposed to be purely descriptive but actually, it profoundly affects the person who is diagnosed. Annemarie Jutel and Sarah Nettleton call for a 'sociology of diagnosis', arguing diagnosis is not only a social process but can be considered an intervention in itself.[6]

Clinicians, researchers and social scientists are already acutely aware of how our diagnostic categories are flawed; that any class is what we define it to be. We are never going to definitively know if some people do or do not have autism. When autism is a moving target, judgement is invoked. Regarding the rise of autism diagnosis, I would argue the question of validity is irrelevant. The more important question than the *validity* of autism as a diagnostic category is whether it is helpful as a diagnostic category. That is, its *utility* should be the focus, not just for clinicians but also for people with autism and their families. The consequence of diagnosis, not whether it is valid, is the fundamental point to consider.

This recommends a pragmatic approach to clinical diagnosis which Jennie Hayes witnessed in her studies, and which was neatly summed up by a clinician academic quoted by Roy Richard Grinker: that to secure services one 'would call a child a zebra' if required.[7] Yet if we unpack this quote it is apparent that being called a zebra is not the only issue; rather, there is a hidden assumption that services are helpful. The deeper complexities of the issue of 'is it helpful/useful?' depend on service availability and whether those services are geared towards doing something that is desirable in the first place.

This begs another question: desirable for whom? For example, diagnosing a child may be incredibly useful to the parent but not so useful to the child. If they are assigned behavioural programmes that minimise their stimming (Chapter 9) or sent on an unwanted 'social skills' programme, as one of our interviewees reported, it may not be helpful as hoped: testimony from the autism community suggests stimming has a useful function in emotion regulation, so efforts to suppress or 'treat' stimming may be misplaced.[8] Benefits of health services and treatments are contingent on the quality of care available and the pathway taken. Calling a child a zebra might yield 'anti-lion protection services' that might not be practically achievable or indeed helpful for the child or her family.

Utility depends, of course, on who diagnosis is useful for, which in turn depends on when the diagnosis is given and under what circumstances. In the next few pages I will consider the functions of diagnoses, who they benefit and the caveats and costs of diagnosis. Regarding whether the rising use of autism diagnosis is helpful, the question of its utility is particularly pertinent to the groups that have come under the autism umbrella since 1990: newly identified adults and children of typical intellectual ability, at or near the threshold, where the bulk of the rise in application of diagnosis has taken place as discussed in Part I.

Institutional functions of diagnosis

Diagnosis is central to the organisation of health as well as social infrastructure and is useful to many different groups of professionals, as well as the people who receive one, as helpfully summarised by Nik Rose.[9] Most obviously, for people with health troubles, diagnosis acts as a gatekeeper to medical services and treatments but can also be key to accessing other services, educational support or skills-training funding. Professionalisation means careers are built around particular types of expertise of a diagnostic category. For epidemiologists and service commissioners, diagnostic categories provide the basis of the prevalence estimates that underlie planning for services. Conferring diagnosis is the core business of a doctor and is what lends clinicians their medical authority. For researchers, diagnosis can serve to highlight areas where research is needed, and research fields and academic journals are often clustered around diagnostic categories. For lawyers, diagnosis can be a condition for involuntary confinement, mitigate responsibility for a crime or confer protected characteristics. For insurance agencies, it is a way to decide who is allowed pay-outs. For commercial enterprises, diagnosis enables the production and development of disease-specific drugs, interventions and the diagnostic tools to identify who needs one.

Diagnosis can also be the banner around which groups mobilise, with charities, support groups and activists lobbying for services and research based on a specific diagnostic category. It can foster a resistance identity that helps feed back into our understanding of the diagnostic category (Chapter 4). For clinicians, diagnosis is a way to categorise and communicate and provide access to services, determining pathways of care and treatment. Diagnosis delineates a set of symptoms for other institutions (such as schools). For epidemiologists, diagnosis may define the outcome against which risk is defined and assessed.

The list goes on. Society's institutions are so thoroughly reliant on diagnostic categories that it is impossible to imagine how they could function without them.[10] These functions can also become vested interests, thereby shaping diagnosis and diagnostic categories and processes in particular ways. Another driver of diagnosis is the infrastructure, industry and professionalism that can grow up around any category. Commercial interests in autism's expansion cover dietary and behavioural therapies but also include aspects of research, education and medicine. This includes the founding of diagnostic assessment services (Chapter 4) and research expansion with billions in funding to develop drugs to treat autism, design behavioural interventions and found glossy, state-of-the-art autism research centres.

Many autism interventions are well respected and established but others are controversial, such as the Judge Rotenberg Centre which until recently used electric shocks to deter autistic children from indulging in unwanted behaviours.[11] Even apparently benign diagnostic tools, such as Autism Diagnostic Observation Schedule (ADOS), are often commercial enterprises that have a vested interest in promoting autism diagnosis, even if not consciously or overtly. Our commentators on the ADOS training highlighted how training is expensive and how it professionalises its services, selling to an elite of well-heeled clinicians and researchers, as well as consistently upselling its products.[2] Commercial concerns can drive the promotion of diagnostic and self-diagnostic tools,[12] and may fuel screening programmes that act as catalysts stimulating rising use of diagnosis.[13] In turn, commercial enterprises loop back to the reification of autism (as a discrete object), leaving it open to commercialisation.[14]

Consequences of diagnosis

I have touched on consequences throughout this book. In this context, perhaps the most important group to consider is the people who are given a diagnosis. A review of qualitative work on the impact and experience of diagnosis for people with mental health diagnoses (published in *Lancet Psychiatry*) shows that, for some people, diagnosis of mental health conditions is experienced as invalidating, whilst for others it validates.[15] Studies reporting on whether diagnosis is experienced as positive find it often depends on whether adults actively seek one.

Being well informed about diagnosis makes it meaningful and gives hope.[16] Diagnosis is more likely to be experienced as harmful when people receive scant information from clinicians, are not told face to face or are kept waiting.[15] Most people find mental health diagnosis validating but it sometimes causes confusion, shock and rejection of the diagnosis.[15] Unsurprisingly, different diagnosis experiences are mediated by the type of diagnosis and how stigmatised any particular condition is in the local cultural frame; diagnosed people report troubling effects of diagnosis, including hostility, exclusion and isolation.[15] Some people report that they are no longer perceived as an individual person but as a diagnosis to be dreaded or avoided. Fear of such stigmatisation led to anxiety about being diagnosed.[15]

These experiences resonate with Bruce Link and Jo Phelan's dissection of stigma via the identification and labelling of differences.[17] Their work highlights the social process that determines which differences are deemed relevant and consequential and which are not. Medical diagnoses vary enormously in the degree to which they are socially significant. Hypertension, bone fractures and migraine, for example, are relatively benign and socially acceptable, whereas lung cancer, obesity and schizophrenia are morally loaded and equated with undesirable features. There is huge cultural variation in social and local responses, as demonstrated by a study which reported diverse reactions to a schizophrenia label in eight countries.[18] This socially significant label leads to the detachment of 'them', the stigmatised set, from 'us' – a divisive process harnessed and reversed by resistance identities for the purpose of challenging dominant forms of power (Chapter 4[19]). A diagnostic label is said to be stigmatising if, once a person is labelled, or diagnosis is disclosed, the person is adversely judged and devalued by the majority. The social response is to isolate, reject and exclude them, which again is a form of exercising (dominant) power.

Clearly, diagnosis can be a double-edged sword, both helpful and harmful. Which edges are sharpest depends on the context and the diagnosis.

Consequences of autism diagnosis

What then can we say about the consequences of diagnosis of autism?

The answers, again, are threaded through earlier chapters but, to summarise, many studies, including one of mine, have shown autism diagnosis functions as a key to unlock numerous resources, including interventions, insurance, self-help groups, services support and financial benefits.[20-22] These include:

- social resources, such as access to support groups, holiday breaks
- health services, interventions and treatments, such as child and adolescent mental health services
- respite care
- access to information (once a condition is identified you can find out much more about it)
- financial resources, such as child benefits
- educational resources, often one-to-one support in class by a teaching assistant or a place in a special school or individual teaching unit.

In the USA, one study showed rates of diagnosis are higher in areas where there is more educational spending and diagnosis was linked to access to a school health centre (rates were also correlated to the concentration of paediatricians).[23] Before 1990, children with intellectual impairment may have been classified as having mild intellectual disability or developmental delay; today, autism is diagnosed in substitution to enable access the additional resources associated with the autism label.[24]

The utility of diagnosis depends on what services, what ways they are useful and so on. Parents in our study and others' reported having a diagnosis for their child was useful (to them), due to this gatekeeping function.[22, 25] But there were also caveats, for example, concerning the deluge of professionals. Some parents reported that a bewildering array of professionals descended on their children,

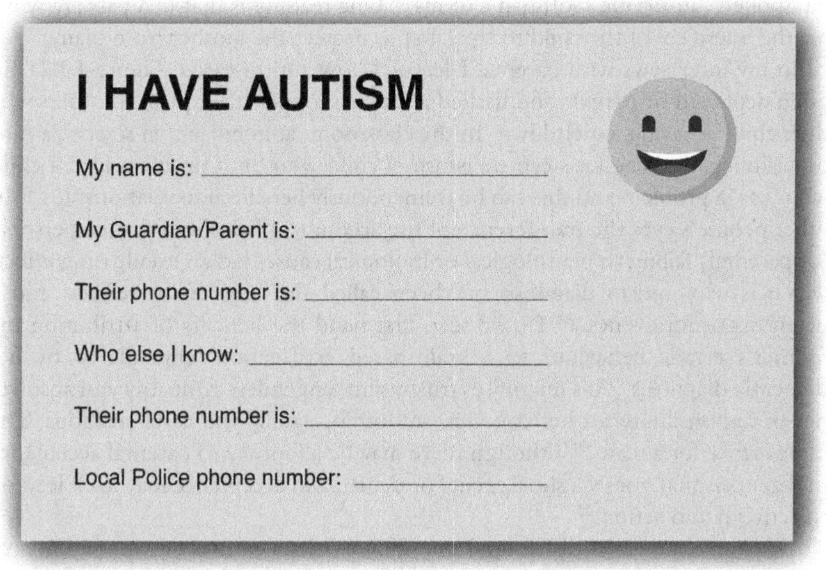

I HAVE AUTISM

My name is: _____

My Guardian/Parent is: _____

Their phone number is: _____

Who else I know: _____

Their phone number is: _____

Local Police phone number: _____

Figure 10.2 Autism ID card.

while others embarked on up to 40 hours of intensive intervention per week (Chapter 2).

Clinical recommendations change with time; what is advised as effective now may be discredited later. The type of intervention considered suitable is contested (for example, Applied Behaviour Analysis), as is what outcome should be its aim: whether autistic behaviour needs to be normalised at all or should be accepted. Some interventions/accommodations remain essential, and their outcomes germane, such as aids to communication, which are indispensable for those who struggle to make their needs known.

That a clinician would 'call a child a zebra' if required also calls into question what the impact of being called a zebra would have of itself. If a child's autism diagnosis is revealed, other people tend to attribute that child's behaviour to an aspect of their brain difference. This transfers a social frame of understanding (such as mother blame) to a biological frame (brain blame). This can be both liberating and limiting. Neurologisation can improve family functioning and lead to acceptance and the setting of that less stringent 'new normal' in expectations of behaviour both at school and at home (Chapter 8).[26]

'Courtesy' stigma is a form of stigma that arises through a connection with a stigmatised person. One study comprising 12 parent interviews showed how diagnosis is crucial for parents to resist courtesy stigma, that is, the stigma of having an autistic child.[27] Resistance to courtesy stigma was achieved by disclosing diagnosis in schools and other institutional settings and supporting a neurological model for children's behaviour. Inevitably, in this process, the child's identity may be 'spoiled', in Erving Goffman's terms.[28] One reading is that in a patriarchy we see the 'sacrifice' of the child to the label to protect the mother from blame.[29]

In my interviews with parents, I learned how autism cards (Figure 10.2) are often deployed by parents and flashed at other shoppers to explain to others why their child is having a meltdown. In the classroom, at home and in society, a card proclaiming the diagnosis can transform a child who 'is' a problem into a child who 'has' a problem and this can be tremendously beneficial to relationships.[30] In other people's eyes the transference of the account of behaviour from a personal (or parental) failing to neurological or biological causes has an exculpating effect, which is why autism diagnosis has been called the 'not guilty verdict' and a diagnosis of forgiveness.[31] I have seen first-hand the benefits of attributing my mother's erratic behaviour to a brain-based explanation, engendered by her dementia diagnosis. This minimises frustration, engenders sympathy and absolves her of responsibility for her conduct, smoothing family and carer relations. The same is true for autism,[21] although there may be a journey to parental acceptance of diagnosis that goes via shock, relief or denial, and acceptance may itself lead on to activism and action.[22]

Of course, power is distributed unevenly. When a card is shown, parents (or those with disciplinary authority) have more power to determine the course of action than the autistic child. For young children, escaping the power is impossible but as children become more autonomous as adolescents and adults, resistance is possible, and even indispensable, to question both being and having 'a problem'. Alternative discourses to autism-as-disorder, other possibilities, other ways of thinking, notably autism-as-identity, have sprung up in resistance.

Responsibility and autism diagnosis

A study we conducted in secondary schools illustrated the shift in attribution of personal responsibility that was engendered by disclosure of a diagnosis.[30] We set up an interactive session with 250 pupils. We provided them with descriptions of three boys in a series of vignettes read out to them by our research team, led by Rhianna White and Jean Harrington. One of the vignettes described Alex, a fictional adolescent who had a strong interest in science fiction and biking. Alex, it was revealed, hated untidiness and felt anxious if his stuff was moved. He was also pedantic, very funny, picky over food and loved *Star Trek* and helping friends with homework. We designated Alex to have clinical-level autistic behaviours, as well as strengths, referring to the DSM criteria to achieve this. Crucially, half the pupils who heard the vignettes were told that Alex had a diagnosis of autism, while the other half were not informed of it. Using a series of questionnaires, we then compared whether disclosing the diagnosis altered the pupils' attitudes towards Alex.

Results showed that disclosure of diagnosis did not alter how close pupils wanted to be to Alex, or how they felt about him, but it did lessen his personal responsibility they attributed for his idiosyncratic behaviour.[30] They were less likely to see Alex's behaviour as being under his control if the diagnosis was disclosed. The disclosure of autism diagnosis meant they were more likely to think Alex behaved as he did because of differences in his brain. This effect – divested perceived personal responsibility for action – has both positive and negative consequences.

Because diagnosis promotes the understanding of behaviour in terms of neurological difference and can sometimes be invoked to excuse transgressive behaviour ('it's not me, it's my brain'), this reading may be associated with loss of the feeling of being in control of one's destiny, instigating loss of power that may be associated with feelings of helplessness. Diagnosis and disclosure may undermine others' belief in a child's ability to progress;[32] teachers, and others, may operate an unconscious expectancy bias because expectations are lowered: they believe that a child is less capable than their peers.[33]

Such biases have been shown to operate in a series of psychology studies over many decades.[34] In one of the earliest and most influential of these 'Pygmalion' studies, researchers posed as educational psychologists and tested a class in school, sharing with the teachers that a fifth of their pupils were 'intellectual bloomers', despite these pupils being selected at random.[35] When pupils were re-examined a year later the 'bloomers' really did perform better in intelligence tests. Once an expectation was set, the authors argued, people – in this case, teachers – tend to act in ways that are consistent with the expectation. The expectation shapes teachers' behaviour, which influences children's outcomes, inducing a new reality.

Expectancy bias is closely related to the idea of the 'autism lens', discussed in Chapter 6, in which behaviours are interpreted in the light of autism. Such a lens allows one to reframe others' and possibly one's own behaviour in an autistic light, perhaps ascribing a lay diagnosis where a medical diagnosis is not given or disclosed. Adults diagnosed with autism are documented to interpret their past experiences in the diagnostic frame, applying the lens successfully and sometimes retrospectively to their own lives.[31, 36, 37] This provides an explanation for a lifetime's experiences of difference. Rewriting biography in this way, often through identification via diagnosis, is known as biographical disruption;[38] 'putting a name to it' has been reported by autistic adults as a cathartic, healing and helpful way to make sense of one's history.[39] In contrast, some adult participants our group interviewed in residential care settings indicated they were totally unaware they had an autism diagnosis.

Stigma

Whether stigmatisation is due to the application of the diagnostic label or to the autistic behaviours themselves is hard to untangle. Our school-based study attempted to examine the effect of labelling while controlling for autistic behaviours, as have others,[40–42] using similar vignettes but such research designs are limited in the ways they mimic reality, as what participants confess their attitudes to be may not marry with their actions. One US study found that telling a child about a peer's 'bogus' label of ADHD meant they spent less time and effort interacting with the peer who had the bogus label. But actually having a diagnosis, that is, not having been identified but displaying traits,[43] reduced the level and quality of interaction more than having the bogus label applied. This type of work is difficult to generalise, as local settings have a massive influence on how the diagnosis is understood and interpreted.

Internationally, understandings of autism vary widely, particularly in developing countries. A London conference hosted by Bonnie Evans in 2017 provided insights from guests who worked with autistic groups from around the world. In Ethiopia, delegates reported, autism is bracketed as a mental health problem and in some rural settings children are chained, enabling their mothers to work in the fields.[44] In Tanzania, the category is not applied to adults or higher-functioning people.[45] In Taiwan, learning to speak later than is typical for most infants (which in the West is considered a sign of autism and developmental delay) is seen as predicting a brilliant future.[46] The Chinese translation of 'autism' emphasises loneliness. In South Korea an autism label is heavily stigmatising, whereas in Australia delegates reported the diagnosis can be a useful mechanism to deflect blame from the parents.

The ways both autistic behaviour and autism diagnosis are interpreted and operated vary hugely among different cultures. Similarly, the relationship between impairment and the social demands put on children varies in different cultural milieus. One the one hand, if research harking from higher-income countries is uncritically projected on to the rest of the world, there is a danger that culturally determined social reactions may be incorrectly interpreted as pathological (eye contact is a good example). On the other hand, a medical explanation of children's behaviour may either be less harmful than competing models in the local setting, such as possession by evil spirits, or can deflect blame. My prediction is that the use of autism as a diagnosis will continue to increase globally, largely because of the efforts and vested interests of the institutions, tribes and individual people that find it overwhelmingly useful and beneficial.

It is safe to say that, since 1990, at least in high-income countries, stigmatisation of autism has been reduced (Chapters 4–7). Autism diagnosis is now not only linked to impairment but also to productivity, focus, breakthrough and creativity. There are stories about famous artists, political leaders and scientists diagnosed with autism (Chapter 6). Advocates with other neurodevelopmental conditions are ploughing a similar furrow; for example, there is an emerging narrative around on the strengths of ADHD.[47-49] These stories promote diagnostic biographies and create a kind of social capital around diagnosis.[50] In this sense, diagnosis is an asset that can be deployed or weaponised to achieve the required or desired ends, which has led to appropriation of diagnostic labels when no clinical diagnosis has been made (see Conclusion).[51]

We made a contribution to the effort to switch focus from deficits in a study mapping how adults with autism experienced their condition as advantageous,[52] arguing that first-person accounts can locate the benefits of autistic people's abilities in real-life experiences. All but one autistic participant in our study described their traits as bringing some advantage, albeit in limited circumstances. Hyper-focus, attention to detail, good memory and creativity were most frequently described as beneficial traits. Participants also described their skills in social interaction, such as honesty, loyalty and empathy for others with autism.

However, the study had a flawed question, in that some participants found it impossible to separate what was 'them' from what was 'autism', in line with Sinclair's pioneering work (Chapter 4). Autistic people described themselves as having behavioural or personality traits but did not necessarily identify them as 'autistic'. Most traits (for example, hyper-sensitivity), were reported as *both* beneficial (to experience the world in all its splendour) *and* impairing (the experiencing of sensory overload). Traits could act as both strengths and weaknesses, depending on the extent to which participants felt they were in control of their behaviour and on the situation. This raised the question of whether interventions targeted at removing autistic difficulties might throw the baby out with the bathwater; some valuable aspects might be lost by trying to treat 'autism' *per se*. A new model to look at autism was suggested, along the lines of a neurological 'shift' in development, with possible positive and negative consequences, rather than the purely deficit-focused diagnostic model.

To avoid deficit-based criteria, and for other reasons, various alternatives to the DSM and standard classification systems have been developed. These include the World Health Organization's *International Classification of Functioning, Disability and Health* (ICD), which includes a list of environmental factors, as functioning occurs in relation to context.[53] In the UK, the *Power Threat Meaning Framework* was an attempt by clinical psychologists to provide an alternative clinical description to diagnostic language[54] and the US National Institute of Mental Health, which is the world's largest funder of mental health research, developed the *Research Domain Criteria*, which attempt to map dimensions of functioning to underlying biological systems.[55] Despite these efforts, the clinical diagnostic framework outlined in DSM-5 and ICD-11 remains the standard set of criteria for clinical diagnosis.

A focus on strengths, or a remapping of criteria, not only simply reflects reality but also builds the language for people to interpret and construct a reality, or an identity, in terms of their diagnosis. The autism story illustrates how a diagnosis evolves in part through the telling of it. Narrative reconstruction involves resistance to dominant ideologies, in this case the deficit-based medical language. to 'suffer' from 'symptoms' or be 'at-risk' in the psychiatric lexicon are value-laden meaning 'less than'; if autism is an identity it is analogous to saying one 'suffers from' and ethnicity, 'symptoms of' a sexuality or 'at-risk' of being female (etc.). Nevertheless, the resistance identity of neurodiversity co-opts the language of diagnosis and prominent activists advocate for further diagnostic expansion. Over time, this contributes to a net shift to de-stigmatise autism and provide a less-pathologising language, seeding a gradual change in public perception, at least in higher-income countries. Advertising, television, books, music and school curricula increasingly cover autism and other mental health conditions, bringing them into the mainstream and promoting acceptance (Figure 4.2).

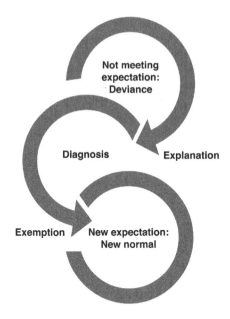

Figure 10.3 How diagnosis transforms the frame of view.

Rhetorically, these developments reduce the stigma surrounding mental health and neurodevelopmental diagnosis and edge them further into the mainstream.[50]

The sociologist Svend Brinkmann describes how, since 1990, autism and other psychiatric diagnoses have been integrated into the cultural artefacts and language of everyday life.[56] The modern diagnostic culture, our eagerness for diagnosis as the go-to explanatory framing of difference, shows we live in *the age of diagnosis*. This is why diagnosis not only occurs in the clinical context but has spun out in the multiple ways in which extra-clinical diagnoses are applied, be it to friends, celebrities, fictional characters or pets (Chapter 6). A rise in diagnosis itself means a loop of increased awareness, which tends to de-stigmatise the condition and leads to more diagnosis. Our diagnostic era and culture help millions but also individualise people's problems, obscuring the context in which their troubles become apparent, coming at the expense of more politically mobilising social explanations or more spiritual explanations.[56]

One last effect of the clinical diagnosis of more types of people as 'X' is the impact on people who do not have a diagnosis. A consequence is the 'shrinking normal', outlined in Chapter 7. Inevitably, diagnosis, when acting as an exemption for unorthodox behaviour and setting a new expectation of normal (Figure 10.3), has repercussions in terms of how non-diagnosed people's unorthodox behaviour is viewed; what non-conformist behaviour is 'allowed' unless theres is a diagnosis to explain behaviours. Diagnosis counts as a form of exceptionalism for aberrant behaviour; an exception is made and judgement is suspended, and a biological attribution for behaviour becomes implicit. Unfortunately, in this suspension of judgement, more pronounced judgement creeps in for 'aberrant' behaviour unmitigated by an official diagnostic stamp, i.e. no valid (biological) impairment.

Dilemmas of diagnosis

Eyal and colleagues' thesis is that the autism category was expanded in reaction to de-institutionalisation and the need to classify children according to who benefited from an educational and structured approach to therapy (which they suggest benefits all children on the spectrum, both severe and not so severe); in their words, all 'atypical children'.[57] This, they argue, was what initially drew a heterogeneous population of children together under the autism banner. However, their point, that for autism the 'abstraction of a category' pulls 'too thin as to become meaningless', returns us to the question of validity. This seems to contradict their point: it is exactly because autism can be so meaning*ful* to so many different tribes and parties that it is expanding.

A pragmatic approach to diagnosis raises the question of who decides what counts as beneficial, rendering the power dynamic between clinicians and patient more obvious; the clinicians decide which people will benefit from receiving a diagnosis and when. Diagnosis may be of more use to the mother than to the child or the father, for example in cultures in which the mothers do the bulk of childcare and may be held responsible for children's perceived failings. Other questions arise: for example, if utility is key, should diagnosis be lifelong or kept under regular review?

Clearly, autism and other diagnoses perform many valuable roles: improving relations, rewriting biographies, unlocking resources and performing numerous institutional functions. Many people have attested that they benefit in many different ways; many people and many institutions have vested interests in gaining something from diagnosis. But the double edge of the sword of diagnosis is obvious to tribes of all stripes. Diagnosis is neither good nor bad, like globalisation. Some aspects are helpful, others less so. The picture is complicated and layered. Autism is a good diagnostic example to study this.

Parents in our interviews experienced dilemmas when weighing up whether to pursue an autism diagnosis for their child.[22] On the one hand, they thought extra resources and support would be helpful, yet feared the impact of a lifelong label. Clinicians wanted desperately to help but described an internal struggle or dilemma.[15] Such dilemmas belie the fact that diagnosis is almost universally promoted in autism literature and for neurodevelopmental and mental health conditions. Researchers, clinicians, autistic adults and the parents of autistic children, and the organisations that represent them, have argued for more and faster autism diagnosis, as the positives outweigh the negatives (Chapter 2). Diagnosis is actively promoted by many of these groups, via policy and personal communications to 'get the diagnosis!', embellished with narratives around the problems of people missing out diagnosis and the rhetorical devices of 'earlier is better', and so forth, that have fired the diagnostic culture of our times. Whether or not the positives outweigh the negatives depends on the context in which the diagnosis is given or disclosed. This is experienced as a tricky balancing act for parents, clinicians and autistic adults.

References

1. Mandy, W. The Research Domain Criteria: A New Dawn for Neurodiversity Research? *Autism* **22**, 642–644 (2018).
2. Timimi, S., Milton, D., Bovell, V., Kapp, S. & Russell, G. Deconstructing Diagnosis: Four Commentaries on a Diagnostic Tool to Assess Individuals for Autism Spectrum Disorders. *Auton. Birm. Engl.* **1** (2019) AR26.
3. Gillberg, C. The ESSENCE in Child Psychiatry: Early Symptomatic Syndromes Eliciting Neurodevelopmental Clinical Examinations. *Res. Dev. Disabil.* **31**, 1543–1551 (2010).
4. Kendell, R. & Jablensky, A. Distinguishing Between the Validity and Utility of Psychiatric Diagnoses. *Am. J. Psychiatry* **160**, 4–12 (2003).
5. London, E. The Role of the Neurobiologist in Redefining the Diagnosis of Autism. *Brain Pathol. Zurich Switz.* **17**, 408–11 (2007).
6. Jutel, A. & Nettleton, S. Towards a Sociology of Diagnosis: Reflections and Opportunities. *Soc. Sci. Med. 1982* **73**, 793–800 (2011).
7. Grinker, R. R. *Unstrange Minds: Remapping the World of Autism* (Basic Books, 2008).
8. Kapp, S. K. *et al.* 'People Should be Allowed to do what they Like': Autistic Adults' Views and Experiences of Stimming. *Autism* 1362361319829628 (2019) doi:10.1177/1362361319829628.
9. Rose, N. What is Diagnosis for? (2013). Royal College of Psychiatry: Conference on DSM-5 and the Future of Diagnosis. https://nikolasrose.com/wp-content/uploads/2013/07/Rose-2013-What-is-diagnosis-for-IoP-revised-July-2013.pdf
10. Rosenberg, C. E. The Tyranny of Diagnosis: Specific Entities and Individual Experience. *Milbank Q.* **80**, 237–260 (2002).
11. Kapp, S. K. *Autistic Community and the Neurodiversity Movement: Stories from the Frontline* (Springer Singapore, 2020).
12. Ebeling, M. 'Get with the Program!': Pharmaceutical Marketing, Symptom Checklists and Self-diagnosis. *Soc. Sci. Med. 1982* **73**, 825–832 (2011).
13. Timmermans, S. & Haas, S. Towards a Sociology of Disease. *Sociol. Health Illn.* **30**, 659–676 (2008).
14. Mallett, R. & Runswick Cole, K. How Impairment Labels Function. In *Theorising Normalcy and the Mundane: Precarious Positions* (University of Chester Press, 2016).
15. Perkins, A. *et al.* Experiencing Mental Health Diagnosis: A Systematic Review of Service User, Clinician, and Carer Perspectives Across Clinical Settings. *Lancet Psychiatry* **5**, 747–764 (2018).
16. Horn, N., Johnstone, L. & Brooke, S. Some Service User Perspectives on the Diagnosis of Borderline Personality Disorder. *J. Ment. Health* **16**, 255–269 (2007).
17. Link, B. G. & Phelan, J. C. Stigma and its Public Health Implications. *The Lancet* **367**, 528–529 (2006).
18. Olafsdottir, S. & Pescosolido, B. A. Constructing Illness: How the Public in Eight Western Nations Respond to a Clinical Description of 'Schizophrenia'. *Soc. Sci. Med. 1982* **73**, 929–938 (2011).

19. Castells, M. *The Power of Identity: The Information Age – Economy, Society, and Culture: 2* (Wiley-Blackwell, 2009).
20. Mansell, W. & Morris, K. A Survey of Parents' Reactions to the Diagnosis of an Autistic Spectrum Disorder by a Local Service: Access to Information and use of Services. *Autism Int. J. Res. Pract.* **8**, 387–407 (2004).
21. Midence, K. & O'Neill, M. The Experience of Parents in the Diagnosis of Autism: A Pilot Study. *Autism* **3**, 273–285 (1999).
22. Russell, G. & Norwich, B. Dilemmas, Diagnosis and De-stigmatization: Parental Perspectives on the Diagnosis of Autism Spectrum Disorders. *Clin. Child Psychol. Psychiatry* **17**, 229–245 (2012).
23. Mandell, D. S. & Palmer, R. Differences Among States in the Identification of Autistic Spectrum Disorders. *Arch. Pediatr. Adolesc. Med.* **159**, 266–269 (2005).
24. Shattuck, P. T. The Contribution of Diagnostic Substitution to the Growing Administrative Prevalence of Autism in US Special Education. *Pediatrics* **117**, 1028–1037 (2006).
25. Jacobs, D., Steyaert, J., Dierickx, K. & Hens, K. Implications of an Autism Spectrum Disorder Diagnosis: An Interview Study of How Physicians Experience the Diagnosis in a Young Child. *J. Clin. Med.* 348, 7 (2018).
26. Chambres, P., Auxiette, C., Vansingle, C. & Gil, S. Adult Attitudes Toward Behaviors of a Six-year-old Boy with Autism. *J. Autism Dev. Disord.* **38**, 1320–1327 (2008).
27. Farrugia, D. Exploring Stigma: Medical Knowledge and the Stigmatisation of Parents of Children Diagnosed with Autism Spectrum Disorder. *Sociol. Health Illn.* (2009) doi:10.1111/j.1467-9566.2009.01174.x
28. Goffman, E. *Stigma: Notes on the Management of Spoiled Identity* (Touchstone, 1986).
29. Singh, I. Will the 'Real Boy' Please Behave: Dosing Dilemmas for Parents of Boys with ADHD. *Am. J. Bioeth.* **5**, 34–47 (2005).
30. White, R. *et al.* Is Disclosing an Autism Spectrum Disorder in School Associated with Reduced Stigmatization? *Autism* **24**, 744–754 (2020). doi:10.1177/1362361319887625
31. Punshon, C., Skirrow, P. & Murphy, G. The Not Guilty Verdict: Psychological Reactions to a Diagnosis of Asperger Syndrome in Adulthood. *Autism Int. J. Res. Pract.* **13**, 265–283 (2009).
32. Fogel, L. S. & Nelson, R. O. The Effects of Special Education Labels on Teachers. *J. Sch. Psychol.* **21**, 241–251 (1983).
33. Darley, J. M. & Gross, P. H. A Hypothesis-confirming Bias in Labeling Effects. *J. Pers. Soc. Psychol.* **44**, 20–33 (1983).
34. Kierein, N. M. & Gold, M. A. Pygmalion in Work Organizations: A Meta-analysis. *J. Organ. Behav.* **21**, 913–928 (2000).
35. Rosenthal, R. & Jacobson, L. Teachers' Expectancies: Determinants of Pupils' IQ Gains. *Psychol. Rep.* **19**, 115–118 (1966).
36. Lewis, L. F. Exploring the Experience of Self-diagnosis of Autism Spectrum Disorder in Adults. *Arch. Psychiatr. Nurs.* **30**, 575–580 (2016).
37. Leedham, A., Thompson, A. R., Smith, R. & Freeth, M. 'I was Exhausted Trying to Figure it Out': The Experiences of Females Receiving an Autism Diagnosis in Middle to Late Adulthood. *Autism* **24**, 135–146 (2020).
38. Bury, M. Chronic Illness as Biographical Disruption. *Sociol. Health Illn.* **4**, 167–182 (1982).
39. Jutel, A. G. *Putting a Name to It: Diagnosis in Contemporary Society* (JHU Press, 2011).

40. Butler, R. C. & Gillis, J. M. The Impact of Labels and Behaviors on the Stigmatization of Adults with Asperger's Disorder. *J. Autism Dev. Disord.* **41**, 741–749 (2011).

41. Brosnan, M. & Mills, E. The Effect of Diagnostic Labels on the Affective Responses of College Students Towards Peers with 'Asperger's Syndrome' and 'Autism Spectrum Disorder'. *Autism* 1362361315586721 (2015) doi:10.1177/1362361315586721.

42. Matthews, N. L., Ly, A. R. & Goldberg, W. A. College Students' Perceptions of Peers with Autism Spectrum Disorder. *J. Autism Dev. Disord.* **45**, 90–99 (2015).

43. Harris, M. J., Milich, R., Corbitt, E. M., Hoover, D. W. & Brady, M. Self-fulfilling Effects of Stigmatizing Information on Children's Social Interactions. *J. Pers. Soc. Psychol.* **63**, 41–50 (1992).

44. Roth, I. Challenges and Agents for Change in the Globalisation of Autism: A Case Study of Ethiopia. https://projects.history.qmul.ac.uk/emotions/events/the-globalisation-of-autism-historical-sociological-and-anthropological-reflections/ (2017).

45. Abimbola Adio, I. Challenges of Raising a Child with Autism in Africa. https://projects.history.qmul.ac.uk/emotions/events/the-globalisation-of-autism-historical-sociological-and-anthropological-reflections/ (2017).

46. Lai Pin Yu (National Yang Ming University, Taiwan),'Autism History in Taiwan 1970–1990'. https://projects.history.qmul.ac.uk/emotions/events/the-globalisation-of-autism-historical-sociological-and-anthropological-reflections/ (2017).

47. Antshel, K. M. Attention Deficit/Hyperactivity Disorder (ADHD) and Entrepreneurship. *Acad. Manag. Perspect.* **32**, 243–265 (2018).

48. Healey, D. & Rucklidge, J. J. An Exploration Into the Creative Abilities of Children With ADHD. *J. Atten. Disord.* **8**, 88–95 (2005).

49. Healey, D. & Rucklidge, J. J. An Investigation into the Psychosocial Functioning of Creative Children: The Impact of ADHD Symptomatology. *J. Creat. Behav.* **40**, 243–264 (2006).

50. Singh, I. & Wessely, S. Childhood: A Suitable Case for Treatment? *Lancet Psychiatry* **2**, 661–666 (2015).

51. Singh, I. A Disorder of Anger and Aggression: Children's Perspectives on Attention Deficit/Hyperactivity Disorder in the UK. *Soc. Sci. Med. 1982* **73**, 889–896 (2011).

52. Russell, G. *et al.* Mapping the Autistic Advantage from the Accounts of Adults Diagnosed with Autism: A Qualitative Study. *Autism Adulthood* **1**, 124–133 (2019).

53. World Health Organization. *International Classification of Functioning, Disability and Health* (WHO, 2004).

54. Johnstone, L. & Boyle, M. The Power Threat Meaning Framework: An Alternative Nondiagnostic Conceptual System. *J. Humanist. Psychol.* 002216781879328 (2018) doi:10.1177/0022167818793289.

55. Insel, T. *et al.* Research Domain Criteria (RDoC): Toward a New Classification Framework for Research on Mental Disorders. *Am. J. Psychiatry* **167**, 748–751 (2010).

56. Brinkmann, S. *Diagnostic Cultures: A Cultural Approach to the Pathologization of Modern Life* (Routledge, 2016).

57. Eyal, G., Hart, B., Onculer, E., Neta, O. & Rossi, N. *The Autism Matrix* (Polity, 2010).

Conclusion

Why is autism on the rise?

The growth in diagnoses of autism can be considered a classic case of medicalisation, which Peter Conrad defines as the process through which non-medical or social problems become viewed and treated under medical jurisdiction.[1] In three ways, the boundaries of autism as a category have expanded dramatically since the 1990s:

1. Who counts as having autism has been extended to include new populations.
2. What counts as being autism has extended to include new types of behaviour.
3. How much counts for the diagnosis to be autism has decreased; the severity and frequency of thresholds for diagnosis have dropped.

The first part of this book focused on the first, and least explored, of the above three facets (as applied to autism). Populations that were not routinely diagnosed

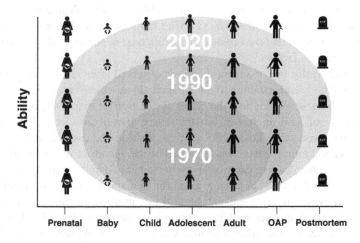

Figure C.1 New populations have become eligible for autism diagnosis as time has passed.

in 1990 include adults, particularly women, children with above-average intellectual ability, and very young children. The expansion of autism diagnosis to these populations (described throughout Part I) is illustrated in a rather schematic way, in Figure C.1.

As the range of signs or behaviours that count as autism has expanded, the severity and the frequency of core symptoms required for diagnosis may have also dropped. As noted earlier, a Swedish study found that, as time passed, noticeably fewer autism symptoms were required for a clinical diagnosis of autism, at least for those diagnosed after the pre-school years, meaning those without very severe impairment.[2,3]. Having said this, our own work on the two cohorts separated by ten years, and indicating milder symptoms might have increased in the UK population (described in Chapter 7) raised for me a question mark as to whether this mechanism was the entire story.

It is not just autism. Across the board, neurodevelopmental conditions have seen rising rates of diagnosis, identification, treatment and accommodations. In high-income countries, including the USA and UK, rates of diagnosis of attention deficit hyperactivity disorder (ADHD) have risen dramatically since 1990, reflected in rising rates of child and adolescent medication for ADHD.[4] The UK and other high-income nations have seen a rise in students' dyslexia diagnoses (at the same time as new policies granting students identified with dyslexia 25% extra time to complete their exams).[5] Rising diagnoses of multiple neurodevelopmental conditions could be taken as evidence for growth in the risk factors that underpin increasing neurodevelopmental traits across the board. Then again, they may be illustrating rises in our diagnostic culture; multiple diagnoses could be on the rise via the three pathways above.

The review of risk factors in the second part of the book indicates it is plausible that a portion of the rise in all atypical neurodevelopment could be induced by changes to some social and medical practices, such as older parenthood and increased births by Caesarean section, perhaps in combination with increased exposure to environmental contaminants.[6] This would result in a rise in autism diagnosis as well as in other co-occurring conditions. Today, some estimates suggest that around half the variance in the outcome of autism could be attributed to environmental factors.[7]

My guess is the rise of autism diagnosis observed after 1990 in high-income countries (the trend established in Chapter 1) is chiefly an artefact of new understandings of autism and the wider application of diagnosis, dwarfing the contribution of 'real' increases, but that there may be an interaction between these two processes. Post-1990 drivers include de-stigmatisation, autism narratives and looping effects, underpinned by the agendas and work of the latest wave of activists, meaning diagnostic discourse has generally become more dominant (Chapter 6). This has strengthened the demand for autism diagnosis. The biggest driver, in my view, is likely the shift in culture towards applying medical labels to oneself and others and interpreting less severe troubles and differences in a diagnostic framework rather than in any other framework, such as the political. We are living through the golden age of diagnosis.

In contrast with the Swedish study,[2,3] our study comparing symptoms to diagnosis through time suggested there could be an increase in the proportion of UK children with milder autistic-type traits, along with an observed increase in diagnosis (Chapter 7), although there was no parallel jump for those with very severe autistic behaviours.[8] As the observed rise has occurred primarily among 'higher-functioning' people, there may be an interaction in which increased risk posed by changing social, medical and environmental practices has increased the number of people with milder neurodevelopmental differences at the same time as they become 'diagnosable'; that is, as the boundaries have shifted.

For example, in high-income countries very approximately 1% more children are now born pre-term than were in 1990 (Figure 8.5). A picture emerges in which the majority of the 'new' pre-term births in higher-income countries use medical technologies such as induction or surgery, are medically initiated or elective and are near term, nearing full gestation. These cases often have neurodevelopmental differences but they are not so pronounced as the differences (on average) for very pre-term children. If what counts as autism has enlarged, people born near term, with milder neurological impairment, may count as having autism. If the threshold of severity of traits required for diagnosis has indeed dropped, then any risk factor (such as near-pre-term birth) that may seed milder impairment may count as an autism risk today, where previously it did not.

Increasingly older parenthood is another pathway that may potentially contribute to a greater prevalence of milder neurodevelopmental difference at the same time as the autism 'bucket' is getting bigger. Such an interaction could account for exponential increases in autism diagnosis (Chapter 1). It therefore becomes incredibly difficult to truly separate the influence of the 'real' from the 'artefactual' in this story, or indeed the social from the biological.

Where is autism located?

Autism diagnosis, despite all our attempts to study it, remains hard to pin down. It seems less like an entity, a 'thing', and more like a complicated assemblage of processes. These occur simultaneously, through time, on many different levels and become something different depending on who is viewing. To take a rough metaphor, think of a pianist giving a concert in a cathedral (Figure C.2).

Autism is identified by diagnosis. Take a moment to imagine that the diagnosis of autism is analogous to whether or not the audience think the music they hear is beautiful. The music is an analogy for autistic-type behaviour; to give a diagnosis it must be recognised as 'beautiful'.

The piano is the hardware of the brain and the keyboard the person's DNA. The make of the piano, its wood, glue and strings, the materials they are made of, and how, is the stuff of neurones, neurotransmitters, the flesh of the body. The player is cognition, conscious thought; the cathedral and organ stool the distal and proximal environment.

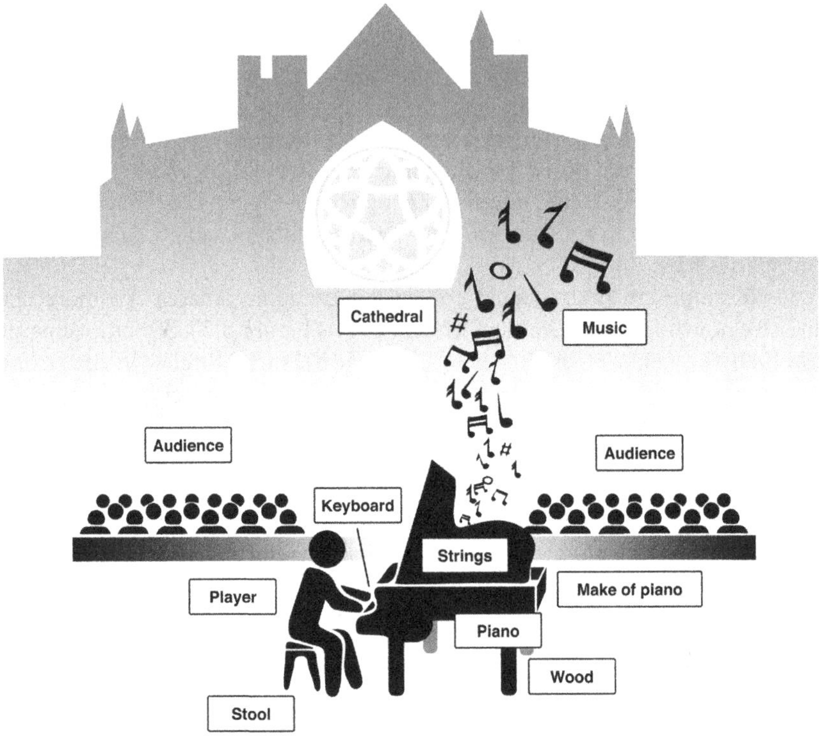

Figure C.2 The cathedral metaphor.

The music the player produces depends on what keys are available. Even if the keys are the same in two pianos, the music may be different. Its tone is affected by what type of piano it is played on, how the piano has been strung, where, what wood was available and local piano-building traditions. Even if the same tune is played twice, the agency and emotional state of the player, how they are affected by the audience (is their partner or parent present?), their hours of practice, will alter the performance; the stool may be too uncomfortable for the player to focus on the notes. The cathedral may be overwhelming or it may be inspiring.

Some in the audience are the clinicians in assessment services who must decide, together, 'Is this music beautiful?', others are relatives and yet others are autistic self-advocates, representing the various neuro-tribes. The same music may be perceived differently by different members of the audience; some may find it beautiful, others may not. The novelty of the music may be a factor. Is the tune ancient or new, traditional or unorthodox? Some may be swept away by the grandiose setting.

Each person in the audience draws on various sources of knowledge about what constitutes good music, perhaps influenced by tribal affiliations. And so does the player. When the clinicians must reach a consensus after the concert some voices may dominate others. The verdict 'this music is not beautiful' may surely affect future performances. And for certain, bad reviews travel. Other members of the audience, who think the music is hauntingly beautiful, may be uncomfortable with the clinical decision. They tell their friends.

Another factor is whether the audience knows the player's desire. Desire for a diagnosis, or desire not to get one, seems to influence clinical decision making.[9] There can be a performative element to autism. That is not to deny many people struggle with, and are challenged by, debilitating neurodevelopmental differences. Of course they do. My emphasis on medicalisation is not meant to suggest autism is not real. I believe that some children develop physical neurological differences and that these can be highly impairing. The reality is that even the most able autistic people experience challenges and often struggle to function.

Autism-as-diagnosed, in the cathedral analogy, seems less a simple construct and more an assemblage of phenomena. Being autistic is seen as located in the piano, discourses of risk entirely locate 'risk' as external or genetic, and autism as the brain-based outcome to be avoided. But the way autism is delineated and officially confirmed through its observation and recognition is impossible to pin down in one place. Autism is revealed as a concept in the minds of clinicians and carers, as a facet of a person's brain, predicted by genetics, neurological make-up and in their embodied behaviours, which occur in interaction with the environment and are mediated by their cultural register, as well as being a product of the evolving history of its classification. Autism diagnosis is a practice reminiscent of what Andrew Pickering calls the 'mangle', the entanglement between the social, material, semiotic and biological that produces and maintains phenomena.[10] Autism-as-diagnosed is an assemblage of biology, society, discourse and the environment.

Today, instead of understanding autism as 'one thing', expansion has meant that, conceptually and in research, people have started to consider multiple 'autisms'. The direction the field is taking is to look at sub-groups, by gender, by age, with and without co-occurring intellectual disability, in verbal and minimally verbal autistic people and in sub-groups by aetiology. There is also a burgeoning field of research on autism-as-identity, at least in high-income countries and, as the neurodiversity movement diversifies and provokes new waves of thinking, beyond autism, this seems set to continue.

Afterword: autism and me

I can't count the number of people over the last five years who have asked me if I am autistic. I certainly think I might have attracted a label of ADHD, had it been as salient when I was growing up as it is now. But it wasn't. I never thought I qualified as having autism. Friends, students, several professional colleagues and family members, even my sister, have asked me: 'do you have Asperger's?' Is this because I work in the field or because of my quirky ways? My partner has often 'accused' me of being autistic, which was not intended as a compliment. He and

I both took the Autism Quotient test; he had a higher autism score than I did. Perhaps I should now attribute his need to categorise me as autistic to his own autistic traits?

People love diagnosis because they need a reason and seem to hate the uncertainty of not naming a difference. I wonder why people seem to need, or want, to attach the label to me. I wonder if they need a reason why I am working on this topic, a personal connection. Perhaps in this diagnostic age, all odd or eccentric behaviour must be classified; we seem to be less tolerant of deviance without a diagnosis, or a name, than we previously were. Lack of a name breeds uncertainty and uncertainty breeds anxiety.

I can't say I have/have not got autism because I do not know what a multidisciplinary team would make of me. Even if they reached a conclusion, I might (like some of our participants) not agree with it. I only know I don't want a diagnosis. The likelihood of me rocking up at an assessment centre any time soon is zero. My difficulties, such as they are, are not going to be mitigated by receiving a diagnosis. Many adults find a new diagnosis to be helpful, almost necessary for them to have an authentic voice in the arena and enable a diagnostic frame of understanding. But is not for me. I would rather the potential explanations were widened to include the political, spiritual and especially the existential explanations covered in Chapter 6, for the loosening of possibilities for neurodiversity.

Before about seven years ago, nobody, anywhere, had ever asked me the question: 'are you autistic?' Twenty years ago, probably no one would have ever asked any academic this question. It is not the answer to the question but the newly minted *frequency* of its asking that succinctly illustrates the points raised in this book. I have not changed or somehow become more autistic over the years. Autism has come towards me. *I have not changed but autism itself is changing and it may soon encompass people like me.* People's understandings of what comprises autism have shifted and people like me, older women, have come to be included in, been absorbed by – and many have embraced – the expanding definition.

I think if I did pursue diagnosis, being near the threshold, if diagnosed I would contribute to the 'shrinking normal'. The march of medicalisation means that, as the boundary around the type of person considered to be diagnosable is loosened, the boundary around who and what counts as being non-diagnosable is tightened. Applying a diagnosis more often and to a wider set of behaviours, to explain deviance, means collateral damage to what counts as *non-deviant* as it is reduced in its scope.

In writing this book, I have come to realise that the language of each discipline, psychiatric, advocacy, policy, even sociology, in fact all texts has an impact on the world in terms of constraining or expanding possibilities for thought and action. The research I have done in the past has fitted in to prevailing discourses where they are published. For example, we recently worked on an article published in the psychiatric literature on *barriers* to medication for children with ADHD.[11] Interestingly, the findings suggested girls are less likely to receive ADHD medication than boys, even when they have equally *severe symptoms* of ADHD, maybe because of *conduct problems* of boys (my italics). My point is that our chosen language, aligned to its discipline, shaped the possibilities of reading this text. *Barriers* suggests that medication is appropriate or needed, *symptoms* immediately frames ADHD as a medical disorder and *conduct problems* suggests that boys have nothing to be angry about or at least that frequent expressions or outbursts of anger are pathological. It is hard to escape the disciplinary infrastructure, yet the example underlines how important it is to have an overview of the flux and flow of knowledge, practices of science and use of narrative and other devices in shaping our understandings without losing sight that many people do have neurodevelopmental impairment which may have a profound effect on their ability to function, and that support is required.

Even the act of writing about a category, like this text, reifies it and pushes it as a framework of understanding. Just as diagnosis is performative, so is my writing about diagnosis. This book is itself performative. Like diagnosis, my words construct an alternative or counter-reality to that enacted by expanding diagnosis. I hope it is one which encourages richer possibilities of neuro-being and relationships. My hope is that this text, if anybody actually reads it, will work towards the expansion of the normal, the standing up for eccentricity, oddness, extreme thought and action as challenging, unexplained and sometimes great, and providing more options for ways of being without resorting to diagnosis. Whilst acknowledging that autism and other neurodevelopmental states entail a different way of functioning, and some people can't communicate, dress, eat and so on without assistance, so people do need services and support, and diagnosis releases these. A line must be drawn somewhere; the questions are where, why, and in whose interests the direction of the line is shifting.

In a sense, our research has conducted a social diagnosis of neurological diagnosis and, as with all diagnostic processes, one of the outcomes is the shifting not only of the 'entity' being diagnosed but of the world in which 'it' is embedded.[12] As diagnosis is used more often to explain behaviours that were previously thought to be part of normal social behaviour, the price is a restricted definition of what counts as acceptable behaviour without diagnosis. I would rather see the normal expanded and new-wave neurodiversity include all people who regard themselves as in some way neurologically 'different', whether diagnosed or not.

References

1. Conrad, P. *The Medicalization of Society: On the Transformation of Human Conditions into Treatable Disorders* (JHU Press, 2008).
2. Arvidsson, O., Gillberg, C., Lichtenstein, P. & Lundström, S. Secular Changes in the Symptom Level of Clinically Diagnosed Autism. *J. Child Psychol. Psychiatry* 59, 744–751 (2018).
3. Lundström, S., Reichenberg, A., Anckarsäter, H., Lichtenstein, P. & Gillberg, C. Autism Phenotype Versus Registered Diagnosis in Swedish Children: Prevalence Trends over 10 Years in General Population Samples. *BMJ* 350 0959–8138 (2015).
4. Collishaw, S. Annual Research Review: Secular Trends in Child and Adolescent Mental Health. *J. Child Psychol. Psychiatry* 56, 370–393 (2015).

5. Ryder, D. & Norwich, B. UK Higher Education Lecturers' Perspectives of Dyslexia, Dyslexic Students and Related Disability Provision. *J. Res. Spec. Educ. Needs* **19**, 161–172 (2019).

6. Modabbernia, A., Velthorst, E. & Reichenberg, A. Environmental Risk Factors for Autism: An Evidence-based Review of Systematic Reviews and Meta-analyses. *Mol. Autism* **8**(13) (2017) eCollection 2017.

7. Sandin, S. *et al.* The Familial Risk of Autism. *JAMA* **311**, 1770–1777 (2014).

8. Russell, G., Collishaw, S., Golding, J., Kelly, S. E. & Ford, T. Changes in Diagnosis Rates and Behavioural Traits of Autism Spectrum Disorders Over Time. *BJPsych Open* 1(2), 110–115 (2015). doi:10.1192/bjpo.bp.115.000976

9. Hayes, J. Drawing a Line in the Sand: Autism Diagnosis as Social Process. PhD thesis. https://ore.exeter.ac.uk/repository/bitstream/handle/10871/120580/HayesJ. pdf?sequence=1&isAllowed=y (2020).

10. Pickering, A. *The Mangle of Practice: Time, Agency, and Science* (University of Chicago Press, 1995).

11. Russell, A. E., Ford, T. & Russell, G. Barriers and Predictors of Medication Use for Childhood ADHD: Findings from a UK Population-representative Cohort. *Soc. Psychiatry Psychiatr. Epidemiol.* **54**, 1555–1564 (2019).

12. Lister, T. *What's in a Label? An Exploration of How People Acquire the Label 'Autistic' in Adulthood and the Consequences of Doing So* (University of Exeter, 2020).

Index

Printed in the United States
by Baker & Taylor Publisher Services